Second Edition

Manipal Manual of Emergency Medicine and Critical Care

- Medical Emergencies
- Treatment of Serious Infections
- Basic Approach to Patient Care

"Life is short and the art of medicine is long, opportunity is fleeting, judgement difficult and experience dangerous. The physician must do the right thing at the right time."

— Hippocrates

Second Edition

Manipal Manual of Emergency Medicine and Critical Care

- Medical Emergencies
- Treatment of Serious Infections
- Basic Approach to Patient Care

Sudha Vidyasagar MD
Head, Department of Medicine
Voluntary Health Services Hospital
Chennai, Tamil Nadu
Former Professor and Head
Department of Medicine
Kasturba Medical College
Manipal Academy of Higher Education
Manipal, India

Raviraja V Acharya MD, DNB, FRCP (Edin)
Professor and Head
Department of Medicine
Kasturba Medical College
Manipal Academy of Higher Education
Manipal, India

CBSPD

CBS Publishers & Distributors Pvt Ltd
New Delhi • Bengaluru • Chennai • Kochi • Kolkata • Lucknow • Mumbai
Gujarat • Hyderabad • Jharkhand • Nagpur • Patna • Pune • Uttarakhand

Second Edition

Manipal Manual of **Emergency Medicine and Critical Care**

- Medical Emergencies
- Treatment of Serious infections
- Basic Approach to Patient Care

ISBN: 978-93-5466-916-3

Second Edition: 2025

Reprint: 2025, 2026, **2027**

First Edition: 2023

Published by Satish Kumar Jain and produced by Varun Jain for

CBS Publishers and Distributors Pvt Ltd

4819/XI Prahlad Street, 24 Ansari Road, Daryaganj, New Delhi 110 002, India.

Ph: 011-23289259, 23266838 Website: www.cbspd.com e-mail: delhi@cbspd.com;

Corporate Office: 204 FIE, Industrial Area, Patparganj, Delhi 110 092, India

Ph: 011-4934 4934 Fax: 011-4934 4935 e-mail: publishing@cbspd.com; publicity@cbspd.com

Branches

- **Bengaluru:** Seema House 2975, 17th Cross, K.R. Road, Banasankari 2nd Stage, Bengaluru 560 070, Karnataka, India
  Ph: +91-80-26771678/79 Fax: +91-80-26771680 e-mail: bangalore@cbspd.com
- **Chennai:** 18/8B, Subbarayan Street, Shenoy Nagar, Chennai 600 030, Tamil Nadu, India
  Ph: +91-44-42032115, 26681266 e-mail: chennai@cbspd.com
- **Kochi:** 42/1325, 36, Power House Road, Opposite KSEB, Kochi-682 018, Kerala, India.
  Ph: +91-484-4059061-67 Fax: +91-484-4059065 e-mail: kochi@cbspd.com
- **Kolkata:** 147, Hind Ceramics Compound, 1st Floor, Nilgunj Road, Belghoria, Kolkata-700 056, West Bengal, India
  Ph: +91-33-25633055–56 e-mail: kolkata@cbspd.com
- **Lucknow:** Basement, Khushnuma Complex, 7-Meerabai Marg (Behind Jawahar Bhawan), Lucknow-226 001, Uttar Pradesh, India.
  Ph: +91-522-4000032 e-mail:tiwari.lucknow@cbspd.com
- **Mumbai:** PWD Shed, Gala No. 25/26, Ramchandra Bhatt Marg, Next to JJ Hospital Gate No. 2, Opp Union Bank of India, Noorbaug, Mumbai-400009, Maharashtra, India
  Ph: +91-22-66661880, 66661889 e-mail: mumbai@cbspd.com

Representatives

• **Gujarat** • **Hyderabad** • **Jharkhand** • **Nagpur** • **Patna** • **Pune** • **Uttarakhand**

For trade terms please contact customercare@cbspd.com

For general enquiries please contact info@cbspd.com

Printed at: Goyal Offset Works Pvt Ltd., Kundli, Sonipat (HR)

Preface to the Second Edition

In a world where medical knowledge keeps increasing in volume and content, wading through information is tough. In an emergency, junior doctors do not have the time to search available literature. Perhaps that is where a book which gives valuable tips at diagnosis, and concise management protocols based on current evidence is welcomed. *Manipal Manual of Emergency Medicine and Citical Care*, positions itself in this area, as a very useful resource.

The success of the first edition of *Manipal Manual of Emergency Medicine and Critical Care* has been very encouraging, as we are publishing the second edition, within a year. This is a testimony to the popularity of the book among students and practitioners alike, and as authors, we are delighted that our book has been widely accepted.

This edition, contains a few minor corrections and additions, which we thought will bring more clarity to the material presented. The format of the book, the topic and chapter divisions have been retained, keeping in mind, the need for it to be a ready reference book.

We are immensely grateful to the support given to this book by the medical fraternity and students, and will continue to strive to present relevant and recent content in future editions too. Your comments and criticisms will help to improve our quality, and please send them to manipal.medicus@gmail.com.

Sudha Vidyasagar
Raviraja V Acharya

Preface to the First Edition

It has been a long time since the first edition of the *Manipal Medical Manual* was prepared and published. This book was designed as a pocketbook for residents containing easy to access doses of emergency drugs, formulae and information needed to manage critically ill patients. The book proved to be a huge success among the residents, practitioners and young doctors training in medicine.

In the subsequent editions, relevant content about usage of antibiotics and management of common infections was added. *Manipal Medical Manual* was never an attempt to replace any of the standard reference or textbooks in medicine, but it was unique as a handy ready-reference guide for doctors at the points of care, in emergency triage, critical care units and internal medicine wards.

We brought out four editions of this extremely popular book. They were revised periodically and reprinted over the last 18 years. The subsequent decades have witnessed a knowledge explosion in an exponential manner, mainly due to the widespread availability of vast information on the internet. The practice of medicine had also become fully evidence-based with guidelines from all major organizations in the world.

In tune with the changing times, we have decided to bring out an entirely new book entitled *Manipal Manual of Emergency Medicine and Critical Care*. This book addresses management of emergencies and issues in critical care, bringing an up-to-date information on the current clinical practices.

The first part of text deals with medical emergencies and related topics which have been classified under headings of various systems such as cardiology (Sec.1), neurology (Sec. 2), respiratory system (Sec. 3), gastroenterology (Sec. 4), nephrology (Sec. 5), endocrine (Sec. 6) and shock (Sec. 7).

In keeping with the unprecedented advancements in medical therapy which have taken place since the beginning of this century, several chapters have been completely rewritten. The management of vascular emergencies such as cerebrovascular accident, STEMI and NSTEMI have been updated based on the current guidelines and recommendations. New chapters have been added such as septic shock (Ch. 54), atrial fibrillation (Ch. 8), tumour lysis syndrome (Ch. 84), Guillain-Barré syndrome (Ch. 20) and paraquat poisoning (Ch. 70), to name a few.

Section 8, which deals with infections (Chs 56–67), has been updated and redone including the dosage of newer antibiotics and their rational use, based on the organisms causing the infection. New chapters, such as necrotizing fasciitis and staphylococcal bacteremia have been added.

Chapters on poisoning (Sec. 9, Chs 68–83) have been made more comprehensive and compliant with current guidelines.

Section 10 includes miscellaneous chapter (Chs 84–87) adding informative value to book.

This book is primarily aimed at the undergraduate students, interns, and postgraduates students to serve as a quick reference guide in the wards, emergency and critical care units. It will also serve as a handy reference for busy practising physicians. We have maintained a simple and reader-friendly approach, as in the previous editions, which will retain its ready-to-use reference value.

The success of the first edition of manipal manual of emergency medicine and critical care has been very encouraging, as we are publishing the second edition, within a year. This is a testimony to the popularity of the book among students and practitioners alike,and as authors we are delighted that our book has been widely accepted. This edition, contains a few minor corrections and additions ,which we thought will bring more clarity to the material presented.

We hope that this book will assist the clinicians in the better management of patients and improve the quality of care imparted. This is the ultimate aim of every good doctor, and the healthcare delivery system. We really look forward to comments, suggestions and criticism to further improve the quality of this book in its future editions.
Please feel free to email your comments to manipal.medicus@gmail.com.

Sudha Vidyasagar
Raviraja V Acharya

Acknowledgements

We are grateful to the continuous encouragement and feedback from our readers across the country. We would like to sincerely thank our colleagues and students for their extremely useful suggestions, feedback and constructive criticism.

Over the last two decades, this manual has emerged from a small pocket handbook to the comprehensive present version, purely by the support and encouragement of readers. We would like to place on record, the contribution provided to earlier editions by Dr Vinod Krishnan. The current book has been renamed *Manipal Manual of Emergency Medicine and Critical Care*, keeping in mind the completely revised contents presented.

The book revision began in July 2019, when some residents suggested that though the book was still useful, it needed a thorough revision in keeping with the tremendous advancements in medical care over the last two decades. The revision began as an academic exercise with the postgraduates from Kasturba Medical College, Manipal: Dr Aaditya, Dr Anisha, Dr Vishal and Dr Pragadeesh, who started the process of editing older versions of various chapters to bring them uptodate, and adding new chapters to various sections. Several postgraduates including Dr Afees Ahmad, Dr Fahad, Dr Tanmay, Dr Vishwajeet, and Dr Pruthvi Reddy edited sections for errors and added relevant content. It is the enthusiasm and commitment of these young doctors that gave us the courage to undertake the painstaking task of revising the book. Dr Nanda Krishna helped in reading and correcting several chapters while Dr Sudhakar edited the cardiology section. Dr Madhav Hande, Dr Praveen Trilangi, Dr Hariharan Regunath and Dr Sanket Shah gave valuable suggestions. We place on record our gratitude for their enthusiasm and effort.

We would also like to express our sincere thanks to publishers CBS Publishers & Distributors for their constant support and ensuring high quality of publication.

Sudha Vidyasagar
Raviraja V Acharya

Principles of Clinical Medicine

1. Common things occur commonly
2. Always think of uncommon presentation of common conditions rather than common presentation of uncommon conditions
3. If what you are doing is working, keep on doing it
4. If what you are doing is not working, stop doing it
5. Medicine is a science of uncertainty and the art of probability

Contents

List of Abbreviations

5%D — 5% dextrose solution
ABG — aiterial blood gases
Amp — ampule
APLA — anti-phospholipid antibody
ARDS — adult respiratory distress syndrome
BD I bd/bid — twice a day
BP — blood pressure
BT — bleeding time
Cap. /cap — capsule
CBP — complete blood picture
COPD — chronic obstructive airway disease
CT — clotting time
CT scan — computerised tomogram
CVA — cerebrovascular accident
CXR — chest X-ray
DNS — 5% D in normal saline
ECG — electrocardiogram
ECHO — echocardiogram
ESR — erythrocyte sedimentation rate
ET tube — endotrachea} tube
FiO2 — fraction of oxygen in inhaled air
gm% — gram/100ml
GRBS — glucometer RBS
HIV — human immune deficiency syndrome
HS — at bed time
ICSOL — intracranial cranial space occupying lesion
IHD — ischaemic heart disease
IM — intramuscular
Inj/inj — injection
IO — intraosseous
JU — international unit
IV — intravenous
Kg/kg — kilogram
L — litre
LFT — liver function test
mEq — milliequivalents
mg — milligram
MI — myocardial infarction
ml — milliliter
mmHg — millimeter of mercury
mMol — millimols
mOsm — milliosmoles
MRI scan — magnetic resonance imaging scan
NPO — nil per oral
OD I od — once a day
$PaCO_2$ — partial pressure of carbon dioxide
PaO_2 — partial pressure of oxygen
PCV — packed cell volume
PO — orally
PT — prothrombin time
Q4H — every 4 hourly
QID/qid — four times a day
RBS — random blood sugar
RFT — renal function test
RL — ringer lactate solution
RT — ryles tube
RTI — respiratory tract infection
SAH — subarachnoid haemorrhage
SaO_2 — oxygen saturation
SC — subcutaneous
Syr — syrup
Tab/tab — tablet
TB — tuberculosis
TID/tid — thrice a day
U — unit
USG — ultrasonogram
UTI — urinary tract infection

Section

1

Cardiology

Chapter

1

Cardiac Arrest

Cardiac arrest refers to the sudden cessation of cardiac activity with hemodynamic collapse. Usually within few seconds of cardiac arrest respiration stops. Occasional gasps may be seen. In primary respiratory arrest or apnea, heart continues to beat for few minutes.

Diagnosis

a. Unresponsive patient
b. Cyanosis
c. Absent breath sounds
d. Absent heart sounds
e. Absent pulse in carotids
f. No breathing or occasional irregular gasps
g. BP not recordable

Golden Rules

- Prompt recognition (each second matters).
- Initiation of cardiopulmonary resuscitation (CPR), and
- Early defibrillation.

Basic CPR—without drug/equipment is also called basic life support (BLS)
Advanced CPR/ACLS (advanced cardiovascular life support)—with equipment/drugs.
For unresponsive, pulseless patient, apply basic resuscitation concepts of **CAB:**

C—Circulation
A—Airway
B—Breathing

Resuscitation should be done by a team, with a team leader who allocates roles to each member. The latest AHA (American Heart Association) 2015 guidelines for advanced cardiovascular life support (ACLS) are:

1. **Recognition of cardiac arrest**
   - Check for unresponsiveness
   - Assess scene safety
   - No breathing or only gasping
   - No definite pulse felt within 10 seconds
   - Call for help

2. **Start CPR** (cardiopulmonary resuscitation)
   - Put hardboard under patient's chest
   - Push hard (at least 5 cm) and fast (100 to 120/min)
   - Allow for complete chest recoil in between chest compressions. Minimize interruption between compressions.
   - Rotate compressions every 2 minutes or sooner, between rescuers
   - Attach monitors—defibrillator with ECG leads and pulse oximetry probe to measure saturation
3. **Airway and breathing**
   - Open patients' mouth and clear the throat of food particle, foreign bodies or vomitus
   - Do a throat suction if secretions present
   - Maintain chin lift position
   - Extend the patient's neck
   - Start high flow oxygen connected to ambu bag
   - Bag and mask ventilation should be started. Extend the neck of the patient. Mask must be tightly fitted over the nose and mouth. Then place the fingers of one hand in the C and E position to secure a seal with the mask over the face as shown in Fig. 1.1. Compress the bag with the other hand.

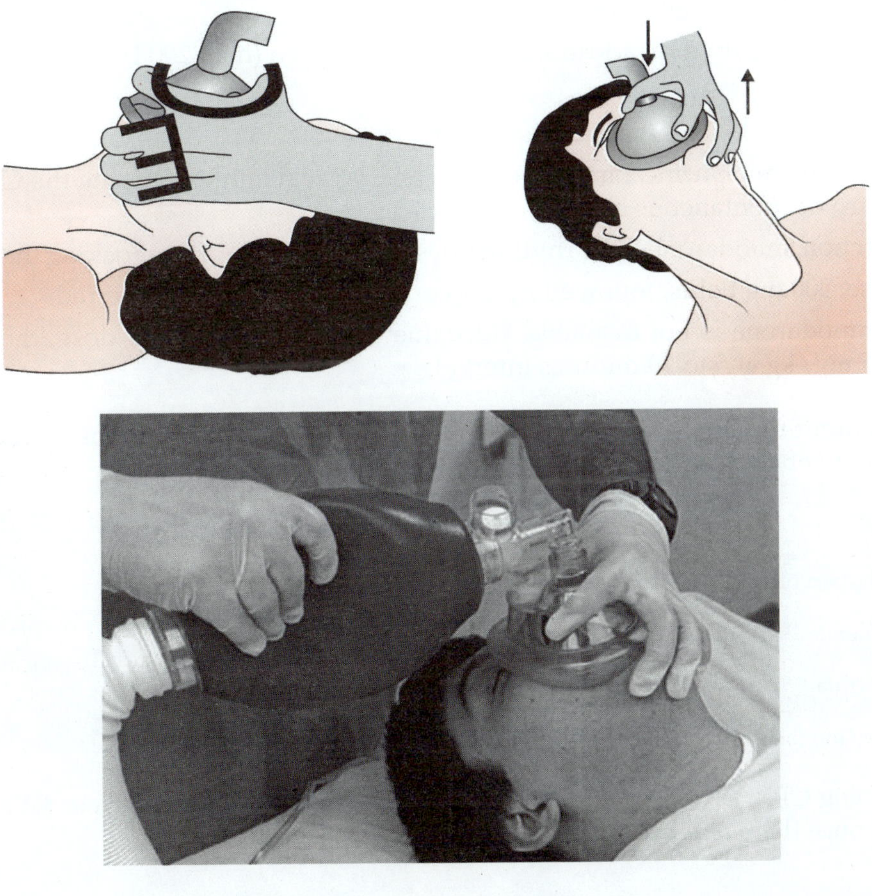

Fig. 1.1

- Breaths to be given in 30:2 ratio—2 breaths every 30 compressions
- Once the equipment is ready (direct laryngoscopy, endotracheal tube (ET) and airway suctioning apparatus) airway is secured with intubation
- Once the airway is secure, confirm the position of ET using waveform capnography. If unavailable, 5-point auscultation can be done. This includes listening for breath sounds over bilateral infraclavicular, axilla and epigastrium on auscultation. Breath sounds should not be heard over the epigastrium, while breath sounds should be heard equally in other areas.
- Once an advanced airway is in place, give 1 breath every 6 seconds (10 breaths/min) with continuous chest compressions.
- Connect the patient to mechanical ventilation (if available)

4. **Analyze cardiac rhythm**
   - If VF or pulseless VT, shock should be administered immediately
   - Initial dose of 120 to 200 J can be given
   - Place one paddle along the right border of the sternum and the other on the left mid axillary line
   - Rhythm should be reanalyzed after every 2 minutes, while chest compressions and ventilation continues
   - Based on the rhythm, additional shocks to be given (max 200 J)
5. **Drugs**
   - A wide bore IV line should be secured
   - Injection epinephrine 1 mg to be given every 3 to 5 minutes during the CPR until return of spontaneous circulation (ROSC)
   - Injection amiodarone if the rhythm does not revert back after shocking the patient.
   - Dose: 300 mg bolus, followed by a second dose of 150 mg if required.
   - If amiodarone is not available, lidocaine 1 to 1.5 mg/kg first dose, then 0.5 to 0.75 mg/kg at 5 to 10 minutes intervals.

While continuing CPR, reversible causes for cardiac arrest should be looked into. These can be remembered as 5Hs and 5Ts:

Hypoxia	Tension pneumothorax
Hypo-/hypervolemia	Tamponade, cardiac
Hyperkalemia/hypocalcemia	Toxins
Hypothermia	Thromboembolism, pulmonary
Hydrogen ion (acidosis)	Thrombosis, coronary

While doing CPR, assessment for pulse should be done after every cycle. CPR can be stopped once there is **return of spontaneous circulation (ROSC)**.

Flowchart 1.1: Cordiorespiratory arrest algorithm 1

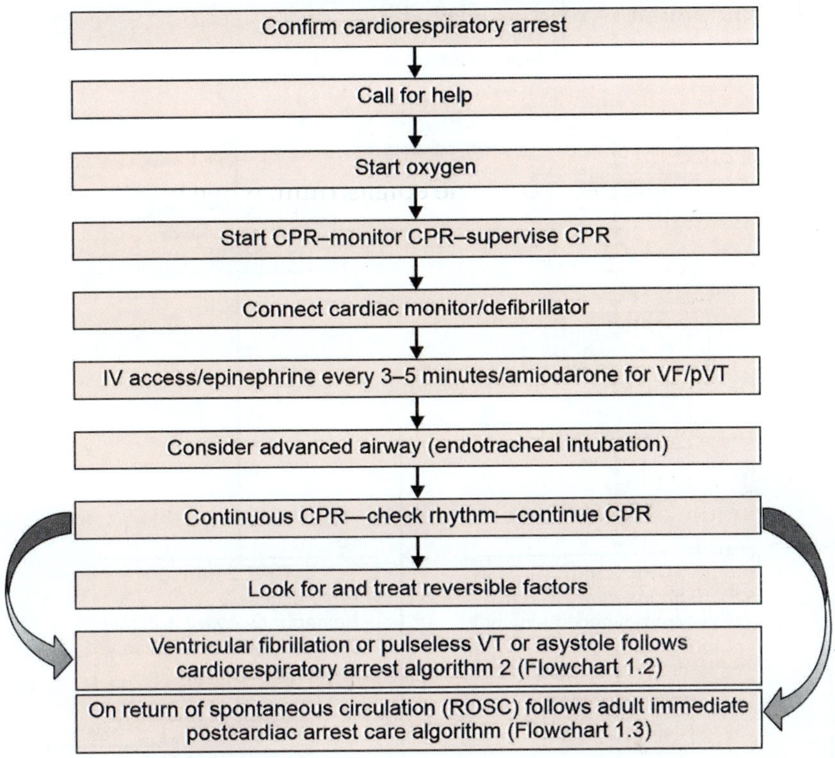

Things required for CPR

1. Suction apparatus or suction line
2. Suction tube
3. Laryngoscope
4. Ambu bag
5. Face mask
6. Endotracheal tube (ET tube)
7. Stilet for ET tube
8. Plaster for fixing the tube
9. Connecting tube between ET tube and ventilator circuit
10. Defibrillator
11. Conductance jelly
12. Cardiac monitor
13. Pulse oximeter
14. IV cannulas
15. IV fluids
16. Emergency drugs (refer to relevant chapters)

Flowchart 1.2: Cardiorespiratory arrest algorithm 2

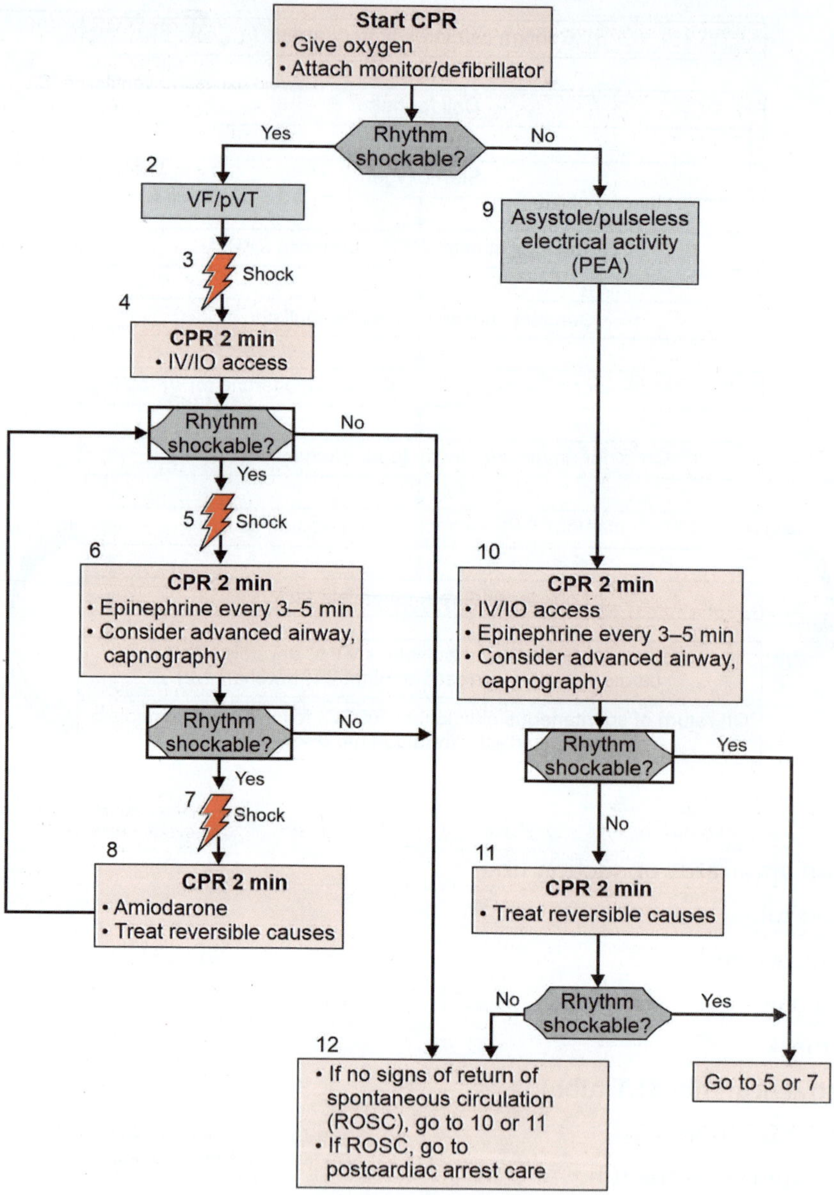

Flowchart 1.3: Adult immediate postcardiac arrest care—2015

1 Return of spontaneous circulation (ROSC)

↓

2 **Optimize ventilation and oxygenation**
- Maintain oxygen saturation ≥94%
- Consider advanced airway and waveform capnography
- Do not hyperventilate

↓

3 **Treat hypotension (SBP <90 mmHg)**
- IV/IO bolus
- Vasopressor infusion
- Consider treatable causes

↓

4 **12-lead ECG: STEMI** or high suspicion of **AMI**

Yes → 5 Coronary reperfusion → 6

No → 6

6 Follow commands?

No → 7 Initiate targeted temperature management → 8

Yes → 8

8 Advanced critical care

Doses/details

Ventilation/oxygenation:
Avoid excessive ventilation. Start at 10 breaths/min and titrate to target PET CO_2 at 35–40 mmHg.

When feasible, titrate FiO_2 to minimum necessary to achieve SpO_2, ≥94%

IV bolus:
Approximately 1–2 L normal saline or lactated Ringer's

Epinephrine IV infusion: 0.1–0.5 µg/kg per minute (in 70 kg adult: 7–35 µg per minute)

Norepinephrine IV infusion: 0.1–0.5 µg/kg per minute (in 70 kg adult: 7–35 µg per minute)

Reversible causes
- Hypovolemia
- Hypoxia
- Hydogen ion (acidosis)
- Hypo-/hyperkalemia
- Hypothrermia
- Tension pneumothorax
- Tamponade, cardiac
- Toxins
- Thrombosis, pulmonary
- Thrombosis, coronary

Procedure of Endotracheal Intubation

Place the patient with neck slightly flexed and head extended (do not in suspected cervical injury). Better to have an assistant and keep all the required things ready and handy

↓

Cricoid pressure over oesophagus to prevent reflux

↓

Hyperventilation with high flow oxygen—pre-oxygenation for 15–30 seconds

↓

Give oropharyngeal suction

↓

With laryngoscope in the left hand, ET tube in gloved right hand pass laryngoscope into the patients mouth, advance to the base of the tongue, identify tonsillar fossa and uvula

↓

Advance till the epiglottis comes into view. Insert the scope between base of the tongue and epiglottis (vallacula) and pull the whole blade and larynx upwards

↓

This will visualize vocal cords. Do a brief suction if secretions are present. (Not to take more than 15 secs for this)

↓

Insert the ET tube between vocal cords and advance till the cuff is just below the vocal cords. Inflate the cuff with air (approximately 5–10 ml)

↓

With the tube in place listen to breath sounds (inflation with ambu bag) on both sides, which should be equal

↓

Fix the tube using either bandage or plasters to prevent slipping after passing a mouth airway

↓

Ventilate with high concentration oxygen. (If patient is restless sedation to be considered using diazepam 5 mg IV slowly over 2 minutes)

Illustrations of Airway Management

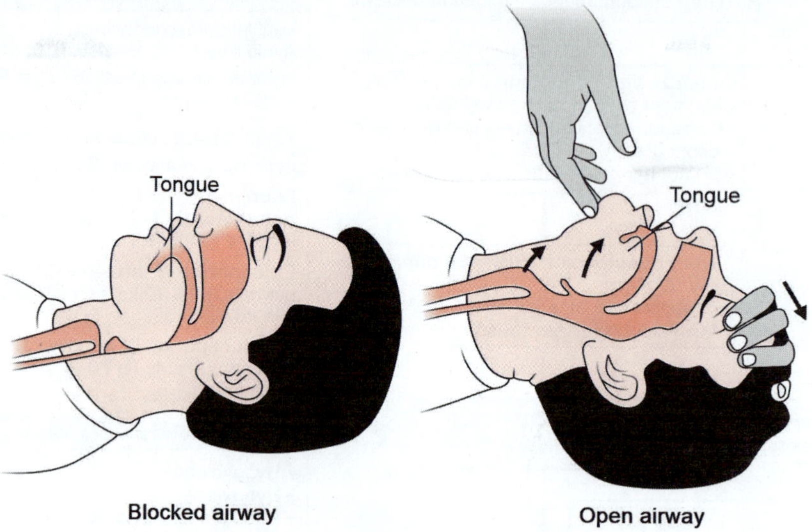

Fig. 1.2: Head tilt and chin lift

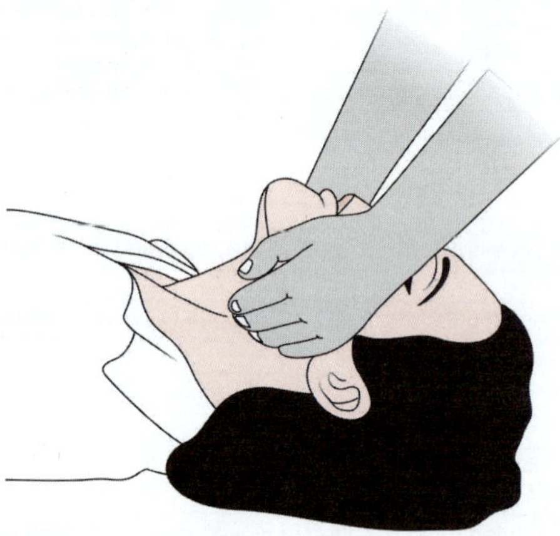

Fig. 1.3: Jaw thrust

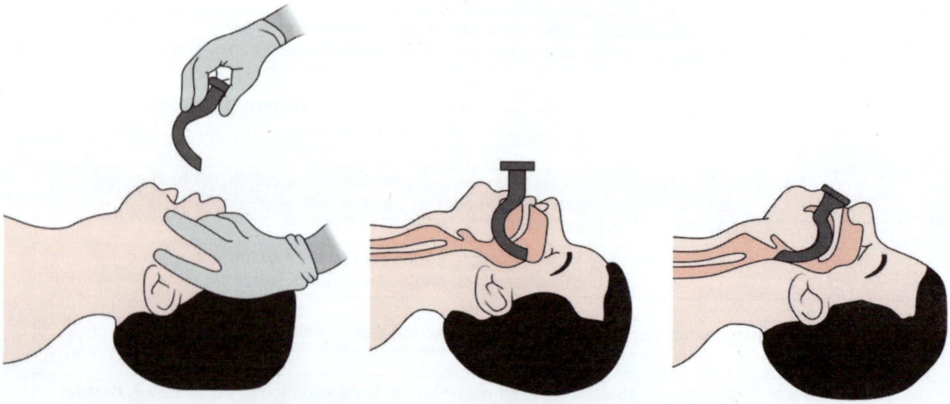

Fig. 1.4: Oral airway insertion technique

Basic CPR

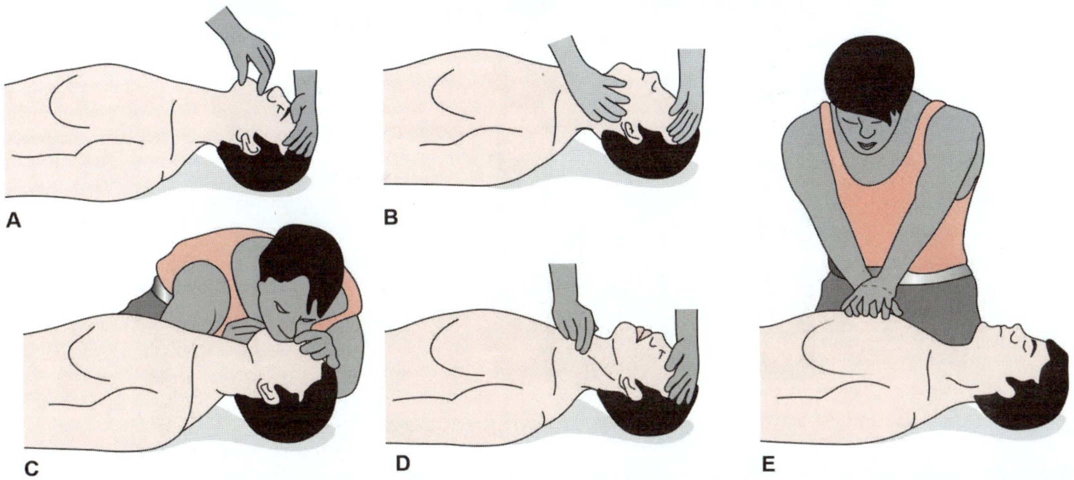

Fig. 1.5A to E: (A) The patient should be flat on his back and his mouth should be checked for debris. (B) If the victim is unconscious, open airway, lift neck, and tilt head back. (C) If victim is not breathing, begin artificial breathing with four quick full breaths; (D) Check for carotid pulse; (E) If pulse is absent, begin artificial circulation by depressing sternum

Endotracheal Intubation

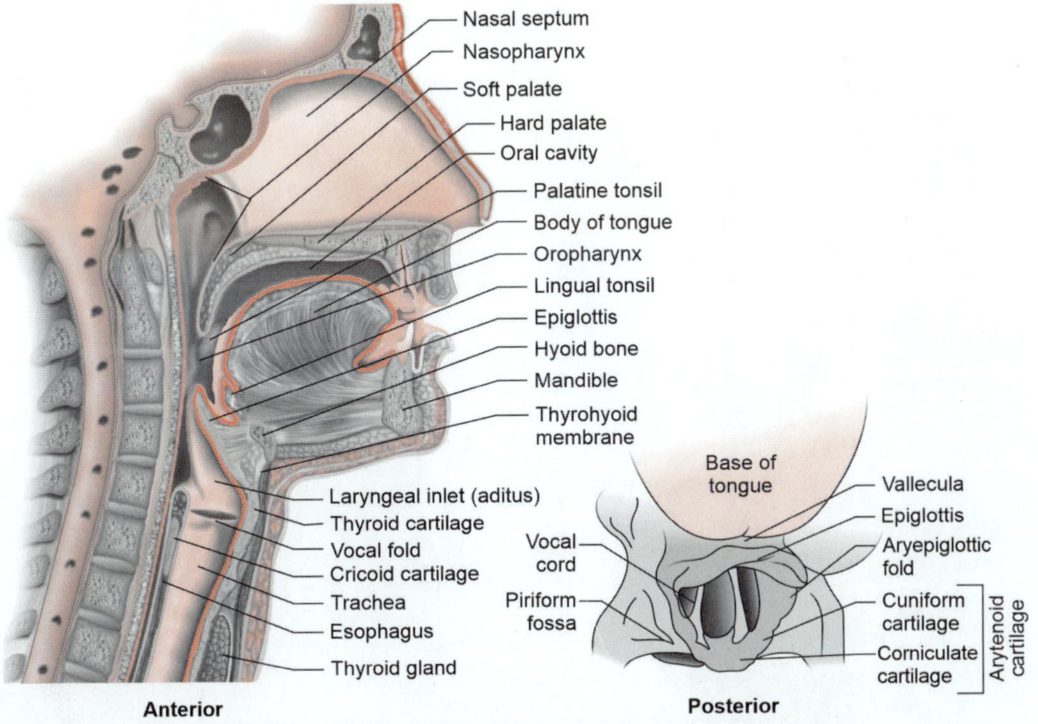

Fig. 1.6: Anatomy of oral cavity and seen during direct laryngoscope

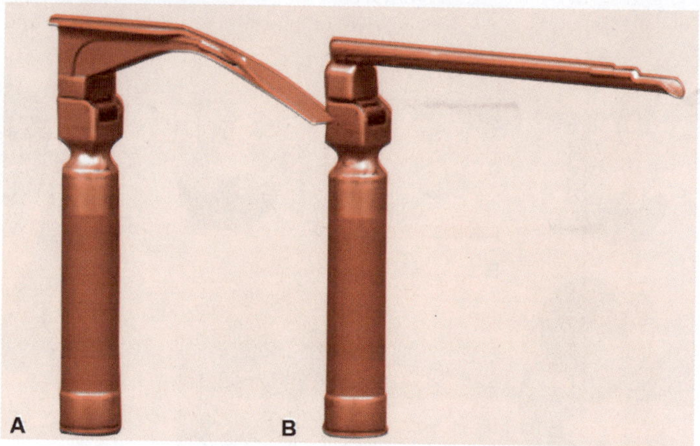

Fig. 1.7: Types of laryngoscope blades

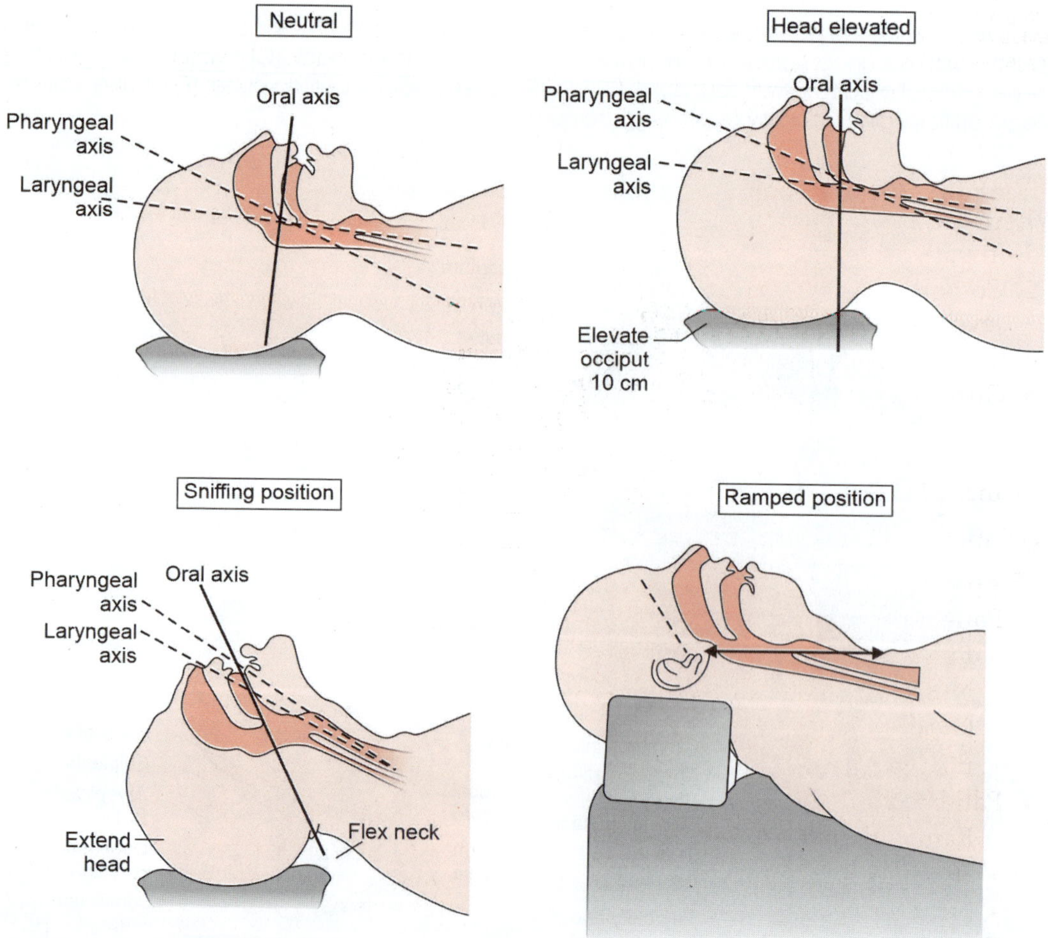

Fig. 1.8: Importance of neck position during airway management

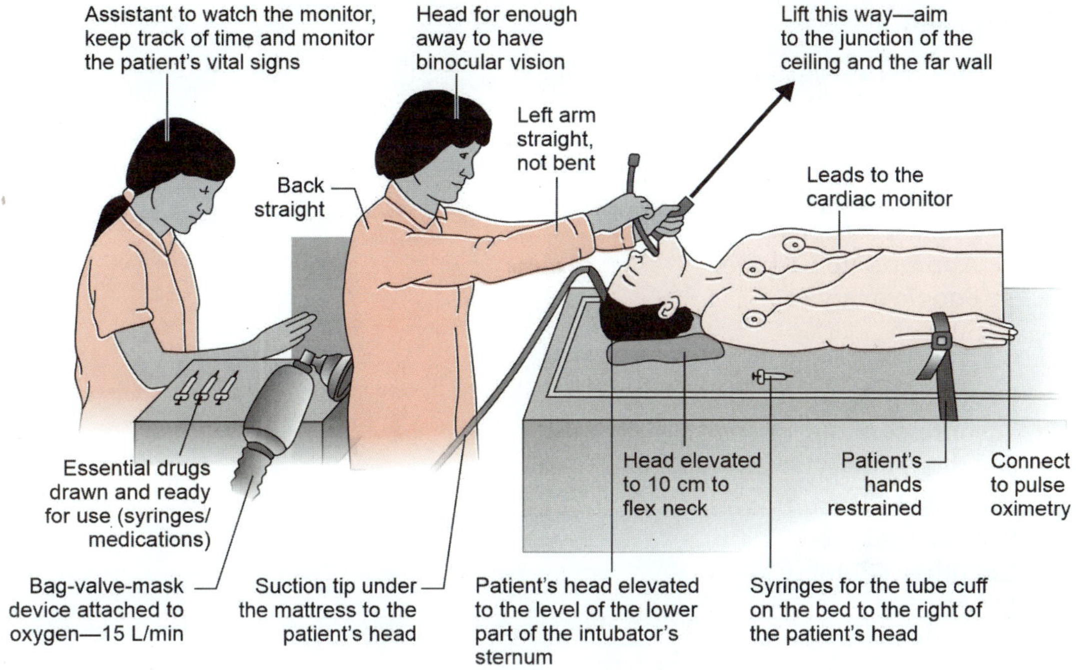

Fig. 1.9: Ideal Intubation scene

Rapid Sequence Intubation

Where it is indicated?

1. In patients who are not fasting or fasting status is not known.
2. Comorbidities with gastroparesis (diabetes, parkinsonism, on opioid therapy, severe pain and gastric banding, paralytic ileus).
3. Gastro-oesophageal reflux disease/hiatus hernia.
4. Gross obesity/second and third trimester of pregnancy/gross ascites.

Emergency Intubation Checklist

Advance planning—periodic review and drills are essential

(A) Patient, (B) equipment, (C) difficulties, and (D) team

A. Preparing the patient

- Patient monitoring
  - Pulse oximeter
  - NIBP/BP recording every 2 minutes
  - Capnography
  - ECG leads and monitor
- Patient positioning
  - Ramping in obese patient
  - 30 degree head up for head injury
  - Neck immobilization for suspect cervical spine injury patient
- Good IV access and fluid running
- Adequate preoxygenation

B. Equipment

- Oxygen supply
- Airway equipment
  - Face mask
  - Airway accessories: connecting tubes, fixer
  - Self-inflating bag
  - 2 laryngoscopes
  - Appropriate ET tubes
  - Bougie or stylet
  - Suction
  - Tube tape or tie
- Drugs for RSI
- Vasopressors
- Sedation/paralytic agents

C. Anticipated difficulties

- Video laryngoscope
- Cricothyroidotomy kit
- LMA
- Difficult airway trolley
- Oxygenation plan in case of failed intubation
- Specific problems

D. Team

- Intubator
- Drug administrator
- Airway assistant
- Supervisor/senior help

Inducing Agents

Drugs	Propofol	Ketamine	Etomidate	Midazolam	Fentanyl
Dose	1–3 mg/kg for patients who are haemodynamically stable. In elderly or hypovolemic patients 0.5–1 mg/kg	1–2 mg/kg	0.2 to 0.4 mg/kg IV	0.1–0.3 mg/kg	2–10 μg/kg TBW
Onset	30 to 45 sec	4 min	30 to 45 sec	Within 5 min	1–2 min
Duration of action	5 to 10 min	15 to 30 min	5 to 15 min	1 to 6 hr	30–60 min
Adverse effects	Hypotension because of dose-dependent venodilation, arterial dilation, and decrease in cardiac contractility	Avoid in hypertension and suspected ICP elevation no risk of hypotension	Risk of adrenal suppression in the first 12 hours	Hiccoughs, cough, nausea, and vomiting, anterograde amnesia, drowsiness, ataxia	Bradycardia, hypokalemia (rare), hypotension

Neuromuscular Blocking Agents and Reversal Agents

Used to prevent coughing, gagging, straining, and vomiting or a patient who is struggling during intubation.

Rocuronium (Preferred)

1. For non-depolarizing agent allows the fastest onset of action and the best intubating conditions, with the least side effects.
2. 0.6–1.2 mg/kg IBW.

Succinylcholine

1. 1 to 1.5 mg/kg
2. Onset within 30 to 60 seconds
3. Adverse effects: Muscle fasciculations, increase intragastric pressure, malignant hyperthermia.

In shocked patients, no adjuncts may be required

Rapid Sequence Intubation Technique

1. Patient should be positioned appropriately for pre-oxygenation and intubation. Sniffing position (atlanto-occipital extension with head elevation of 3 to 7 cm), supported so that the neck is flexed and the head extended-ensure that there is no cervical injury.
1. Secure IV cannula
2. Pre-oxygenation: Give 100% oxygen for three minutes of normal tidal volume breathing, for eight deep breaths over one minute, or until the fraction of expired oxygen is over 90 percent.
3. Give IV inducing and neuromuscular blocking agent.
4. Wait for an appropriate time period or fasciculations (if succinylcholine is used)
5. Open the airway by lifting the chin upward while tilting the forehead back. The goal is to create a straighter path from the nose to the trachea.

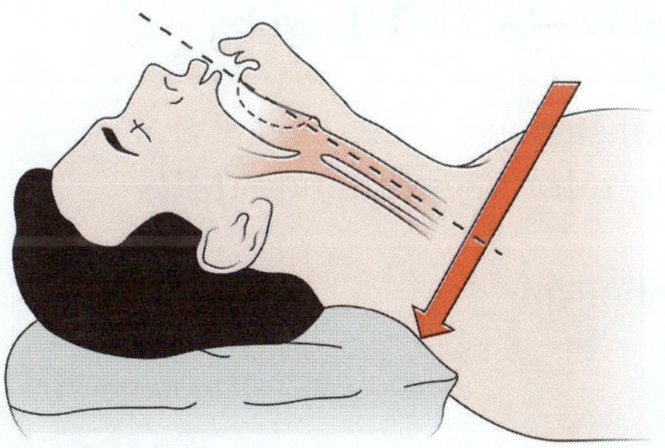

Fig. 1.10: In individuals with a suspected neck injury, the cervical spine should be protected and a jaw thrust alone is used to open the airway

6. If regurgitation is observed, suction should be rapidly applied, and the bed should be placed in a head-down (Trendelenburg) position to minimise the chance of aspiration into the trachea.
7. Once the endotracheal tube is placed, the cuff is immediately inflated
8. Ensure correct position of tube: Chest rise and fall, tube misting, auscultation of lungs on both sides in axilla to ensure equal air entry.

Chapter

2

Cardiogenic Shock

It is a low cardiac output state due to cardiac dysfunction resulting in life threatening end organ hypoperfusion and hypoxia. Hemodynamic criteria are:

- Sustained hypotension (systolic blood pressure <90 mm Hg for ≥30 min)
- Reduced cardiac index (< 2.2 L/min/m^2)
- In the presence of normal or elevated pulmonary capillary wedge pressure (>15 mm Hg), or
- Right ventricular end-diastolic pressure (RVEDP) (>10 mm)

Causes for Cardiogenic Shock

- Acute myocardial infarction
  - Left ventricular failure/RVMI
  - Ventricular septal rupture (VSR)
  - Papillary muscle rupture—severe mitral regurgitation
- Post-cardiac arrest
- Refractory arrhythmias—ventricular tachycardia, ventricular fibrillation, bradyarrhythmias
- End stage cardiomyopathy—DCM/Takotsubo
- Severe valvular disease
  - Critical aortic or mitral stenosis
  - Acute severe aortic or mitral regurgitation (MR)
- Aortic dissection
- Pulmonary thromboembolism
- Pericardial tamponade
- Myocarditis
- Toxic/metabolic
  - Acidosis, hypoxaemia, sepsis

Clinical Features

- Dyspneic/chest pain (angina)
- Appearing pale/diaphoretic/altered sensorium
- Low volume pulse
- Hypotension—systolic less than 90 mmHg
- Hypoxia

- Elevated JVP in RV MI
- Cardiovascular examination
  - Weak apical pulse
  - S_3 gallop
  - Systolic murmurs in case of MR or ventricular septal rupture (VSR)
- Respiratory examination:
  - Bilateral basal crackles
- Oliguria or anuria

As in Cardiac Arrest, Look for 5H and 5T

Look for 5H and 5T

- Hypoxia
- Hydrogen ion (acidosis)
- Hypo-/hyperkalemia
- Hypothermia
- Hypovolemia
- Tamponade
- Thorax (pneumo)
- Toxins
- Thrombosis—pulmonary and cardiac

Investigations

- ECG: To look for acute MI, arrhythmias. Repeat ECG at 2–4 hours if first one is normal and strong suspicion of MI
- CXR: To look for pulmonary congestion, pulmonary oedema, cardiomegaly
- Echocardiogram: To look for regional wall motion abnormality, valvular disease, ventricular septal rupture (VSR), cardiac tamponade/free wall rupture.
- Cardiac markers: Creatinine kinase (MB), troponin T and I, NT Pro BNP
- CBC, RFT, LFT
- Elevated plasma lactate
- Arterial blood gas analysis for hypoxaemia, metabolic acidosis
- Pulmonary artery catheterization (if facilities permit and needed)
- Coronary angiogram

Treatment

- Ventilatory support required for
  - To protect the airway/maintain oxygen in unconscious patients.
  - For pulmonary edema (details *see* chapter on pulmonary edema).
- Haemodynamic support
  - Volume status—judge by clinical and echo findings:
    - If pulmonary edema—give diuretics if BP is supported by inotropes
    - If fluid deficit—small volume boluses of 250 mL can be tried, with monitoring
    - Place central line for delivering inotropes and fluids
  - Vasopressors: Target MAP 60–65 mm Hg
    - Norepinephrine infusion—currently still the first choice.
      - Dose is 8 mg in 42 mL of D_5 or NS (total 50 mL)

- Start infusion at 0.05 μg/kg/min (180 μg/hr for 60 kg person)—around 1–2 mL/hr, then titrate to a maximum dose of 20 mL/hr
- Dopamine infusion
  - Dose: 2 to 5 μg/kg/min initially with maintenance infusion of 5 to 20 μg/kg/minute
  - Diluted as 400 mg in 40 mL NS. Start at 2.5 mL/hr, increase as per need up to 20 mL/hr
  - Adverse effects—arrhythmias, tachycardia
- Dobutamine infusion—add onto norepinephrine if BP is <80 mm Hg, MAP >70 mm, and SBP >65 mm
  - Initial dose: 0.5 to 1 μg/kg/min (0.36–0.72 mL/hr)
  - Maintenance dose: 2 to 20 μg/kg/min (1.4–14.4 mL/hr)
  - Maximum dose: 20 to 40 μg/kg/min (14.4–21 mL/hr)
  - Dilution 250 mg in 50 mL NS
  - Adverse effect—causes tachyarrhythmias
- Adrenaline infusion—add on in case of refractory hypotension and bradyarrhythmias.
  - Dose is 9 mg in 41 mL D_5/NS (total 50 mL).
  - Usual dosing range—0.01 to 0.5 μg/kg/minute
  - Start at around 1–2 mL/hr to titrate to maximum of 20 mL/hr
  - Adverse effect—tachyarrhythmias, increase in lactate levels
- Levosimendan
  - Can be used once BP is >90 mm systolic
  - Dilute 12.5 mL in 50 mL of 5% dextrose, and add to 500 mL 5% dextrose. Run as infusion at 2–10 mL/hr, based on body weight.
  - IV levosimendan is 6 to 12 μg/kg loading dose over 10 minutes followed by 0.05 to 0.2 μg/kg/min as a continuous infusion.
- Vasopressin is the next choice.
  - Dose: 0.03 units/minute
  - Dilution: 40 units in 39 mL normal saline. It can be started at 1.2 mL/hr (0.02 units/minute) and increased to 2.4 mL/hr (0.04 units/minute).
    Management of arrhythmias and hyperglycemia as per guidelines mentioned in those chapters
- Beta blockers should be avoided in cardiogenic shock

- **Mechanical devices**
  Intra-aortic balloon pump, Veno-arterial ECMO, LV support with impella assist device, can be used especially in patients who are being taken for revascularization.
  Indications of IABP: In acute MI in patients undergoing PCI or CABG with
  1. Refractory heart failure.
  2. Cardiogenic shock.
  3. Adjunctive therapy in high risk or complicated angioplasty.
- Fibrinolytics, reperfusion and revascularization for patients with MI causing cardiogenic shock.
  - Further details given in STEMI management chapter.

Chapter

3

Management of Acute Decompensated Heart Failure and Pulmonary Edema

Symptoms and Signs

1. Acute dyspnea, orthopnea, tachypnea, tachycardia, and cyanosis
2. Hypotension or hypertension are common.
3. Pink, frothy sputum
4. Diffuse pulmonary crackles are common; wheezing (cardiac asthma) may also be present

Investigations

ECG: Look for evidence of ischemia, infarction, arrhythmia (e.g. AF/VPCs), and chamber hypertrophy.

Chest Radiograph

- Pulmonary vascular congestion/butterfly pattern of alveolar edema
- Cardiomegaly/alternative diagnoses to be ruled out (e.g. pneumonia);
- Normal radiograph does not rule out pulmonary edema. The CXR changes appear a few hours after clinical picture. The resolution also is clinical first, radiological later (Figs 3.1 and 3.2).

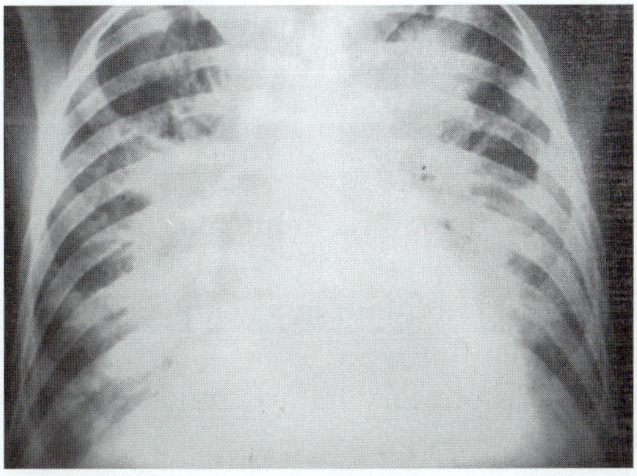

Fig. 3.1: Bilateral perihilar alveolar edema, giving a typical butterfly appearance, with bilateral interstitial edema

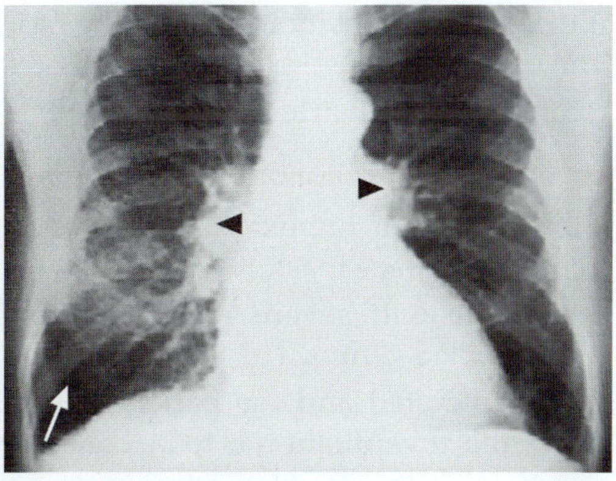

Fig. 3.2: Septal lymphatic distention—Kerley B lines (arrow), pulmonary vascular congestion, and enlarged hilar shadows (arrowhead)

Echocardiography

For ejection fraction, wall motion abnormality, chamber hypertrophy, pressures in chambers, valvular disease and infective endocarditis.

Cardiac Biomarkers (raised in ACS)

- Troponin T: Normal range-(up to 0.020 ng/mL)
- Troponin I: Normal value-upto 0.04 ng/mL
- Serial rise is important. Usually elevated in MI/myocarditis

NT-Pro BNP (raised in pulmonary edema)

- Normal is <125 pg/mL
- >75 years >450 pg/mL is significant
- <300 pg/mL rules out pulmonary edema. Good negative predictive value
- Rise indicates cardiac failure
- Falls with treatment. Used to assess efficacy of treatment
- Values may be falsely high in AF, MI, elderly, and in renal failure falsely low in obesity
- Helps to differentiate CCF from non-cardiac causes of dyspnea

Blood Investigations

- Complete blood picture
- Renal function test/serum electrolytes
- ABG-type 1 respiratory failure
- Troponin T/I: Serial rise is important to rule out ACS

Differential Diagnosis

- Pulmonary embolism, acute exacerbation of bronchial asthma and pneumonia,
- Noncardiogenic pulmonary edema (e.g. adult respiratory distress syndrome)

Treament

- Monitor oxygen saturation, vital signs, and cardiac rhythm.
- Place two IV catheters, position the patient upright, with legs dangling, and monitor the urine output.
- Monitor BP with arterial line, if there is hypotension.

Oxygen Supplementation

- Start oxygen if hypoxic (SpO_2 <90%), preferably through a venturi at 60%/non-rebreathing face mask.
- In patients with severe respiratory distress, trial of non-invasive ventilation (NIV) with PEEP 5–8 mm. This helps to reabsorb alveolar fluid.
- If not tolerated and the patient has persisting respiratory failure, intubation and mechanical ventilation is to be considered.

Morphine

- Very effective in gross pulmonary edema.
- 2–8 mg IV, repeated if needed in 2–4 hours.

- Helps in decreasing anxiety and reducing preload.
- Added benefit of pain relief in patients with angina.

Caution: May cause reduction in respiratory drive and hypotension due to venodilatation.

Initiate diuretic therapy without delay to relieve congestion/fluid overload

- Frusemide 40–200 mg IV (or)
- Torsemide 20 mg IV (or)
- Bumetanide 1 mg IV
- Onset of action is usually after 30 minutes of injection (reduces pulmonary pressure by vasodilatation) and it peaks around 2 hours from the time of injection.

Higher doses are needed

- For patients taking diuretics chronically (e.g. twice home dose)
- Patients with renal failure or severe HF : bolus doses 160 to 200 mg of frusemide, 100 to 200 mg of torsemide, or 4 to 8 mg of bumetanide, OR
- *Frusemide infusion:* 5–10 mg/hr, maximum—20 mg/hr
  Dilution—40 mg (2 amp) in 36 mL NS—1 mg = 1 mL

  In patients with hypotension, to initiate diuretics along with inotropes.

  Once a patient has improved, IV can be converted to oral drugs.

For Patients with Concomitant Elevated BP—vasodilator therapy

- Give IV nitroglycerin in addition (Dose is 25 mg in 50 mL NS)
- Start at 5 to 10 µg/min (**0.6–1.2 mL/hr**) and titrate every 3 to 5 minutes. Based on MAP or systolic BP to a dose range of 10 to 200 µg/min (**1.2–24 mL/hr**).
- ACE-I, ARBs, isosorbide + hydralazine can be used to bring down BP

For Patients with Hypotension

Inotropes

- Refer to Chapter 2: **Cardiogenic shock**

Device Therapy

Mainly in patients with reduced ejection fraction

- Intra-aortic balloon pump counter—pulsations
- Left ventricular mechanical assist devices
- ECMO can be useful

Other Measures

- Bedrest—initially
- Salt and fluid restriction
- DVT prophylaxis-with prophylactic heparin and stockings
- Arrhythmia recognition and correction
- Long term measures—correct ischemia/arrhythmia, ACE-inhibitors, ARBs, aldosterone antagonists, ARNI, beta-blockers, vasodilators
- If heart rate greater than 100/m, consider starting ivabradine, beta-blockers or digoxin
- If patient has associated atrial fibrillation, consider adding digoxin.

Chapter

4

Acute Coronary Syndrome Including Unstable Angina and Non-ST Elevation Myocardial Infarction (NSTEMI)

UNSTABLE ANGINA/NSTEMI

Difference between these two:

- NSTEMI shows **elevation of biomarkers**.
- Unstable angina shows **no rise in biomarkers**.

Clinical Presentation

- **Unstable angina:** Severe chest discomfort—described as, heaviness, tightness, or constriction in the center or left of the chest
  - On minimal exertion, with limitation of physical activity
  - Angina at rest >20 minutes
  - Relatively recent onset (<2 weeks)
  - Crescendo pattern (more severe/prolonged than previous episodes)
- Anginal equivalents
  - Exertional shortness of breath, nausea, diaphoresis, or fatigue
  - More frequent in the elderly, women and diabetics
- On examination—features of angina
  - May be unremarkable
  - Dyspnea—if LV dysfunction

ECG

- New horizontal or down-sloping **ST depression** 0.05 mV (0.5 mm) in two anatomically contiguous leads
- **T inversion** 0.1 mV (1 mm) in two anatomically contiguous leads with prominent R wave or R/S ratio >1
- Serial ECGs at 1–24 hours are important

ECHO: To look at LV function, wall motion abnormalities and valvular abnormalities

Cardiac biomarkers:

- Troponin T/I—serial rise is significant
- Raised in NSTEMI. Not high in unstable angina

For details of interpretation: Refer to STEMI chapter

Other Investigations

- Diabetes workup—blood sugars and HbA1c
- Renal function testing

- Lipid profile
- Hs CRP

Management

- NSTEMI is a spectrum. Can present as mild chest discomfort to cardiovascular collapse.
- Hence it is important to risk stratify patients according to scoring systems and then manage accordingly.

  Thrombolysis in myocardial infarction **(TIMI) score**

Score	Yes 1 point	No 0 point
Age >65		
3 risk factors for ACS: HT/dyslipidemia/smoking/DM/family history		
Use of aspirin in last 7 days		
Prior coronary stenosis > 50%		
>2 angina events in 24 hours		
ST-segment deviation of >0.05 mV		
Elevated cardiac biomarkers		
	Calculate total score	

Low risk 0–2; Intermediate risk 3–4; High risk 5–7

Current Guidelines ESC 2020

- **Very high risk:** Patients need PCI within 2 hours.
  - Hemodynamic instability
  - Cardiogenic shock
  - Recurrent/refractory chest pain despite medical therapy
  - Life-threatening arrhythmias
  - Mechanical complications of MI
  - Acute heart failure clearly related to NSTE ACS
  - ST-segment depression >1 mm/6 leads plus ST-segment elevation AVR and/or V1.
- **High risk:** PCI in 24 hours
  - Criteria are an established NSTEMI diagnosis
  - Dynamic new or presumably new contiguous ST-segment changes (symptomatic or silent),
  - Resuscitated cardiac arrest without ST-segment elevation or cardiogenic shock, and GRACE risk score >140.
- **Low risk:** Patients who lack any of the above criteria, for whom invasive management is selective.

Management will depend on risk stratification

Very high risk

- ASA plus heparin
- Glycoprotein IIb/IIIa inhibitor
- **Early cardiac catheterization within 2 hours**

High risk

- **ASA** plus clopidogrel (DAPT)
- Nitrates
- Heparin or low-molecular-weight heparin
- PCI within 24 hours

Low risk

- ASA monotherapy
- Nitrates
- No heparin
- Observation for higher-risk indications

For patients in low risk with markers negative after 6 hours

- Exercise stress test can be done
- Followed by CT coronary angiogram

Percutaneous coronary intervention (PCI)

- Very high risk/high risk who need intervention must be taken up for PCI as in STEMI. For details refer to STEMI chapter.

Antiplatelets:

- All patients require antiplatelets.
- **Aspirin** is always given 325 mg stat

For those with PCI

- Aspirin (+)
- Ticagrelor 180 mg stat (followed by 90 mg bd)/clopidogrel 600 mg stat (followed by 75 mg od)/prasugrel 60 mg stat, and 10 mg od after that
- GP IIb/IIIa inhibitor

GP IIb/IIIa Inhibitor

It can be used, but more useful, refer to STEMI chapter.

Those not undergoing PCI

Aspirin + ticagrelor 180 mg stat or clopidogrel 600 mg, followed by maintenance doses given above

Note: Avoid prasugrel, if

- Patients age 75 years or older,
- Body weight <60 kg, or
- With past stroke or TIA,
- Bleeding risk is high: clopidogrel 300 to 600 mg is an option
- Prior hemorrhagic stroke, current bleeding, bleeding tendencies, or clinically relevant anemia or thrombocytopenia.

Duration of DAPT

For NSTEMI with PCI or medical treatment is **one year**

Anticoagulation: It is must in all patients

- Anticoagulation is **very important in NSTEMI** and is done with heparin/enoxaparin/fondaparinux.

Heparin

- In early PCI (4–48 hours)
- Dose is 80 IU/kg stat, and run a drip at 18 u/kg for 24 hours, target an aPTT of 1.5–2 times normal.
- Or 5000 IU 8th hourly SC

Bivalirudin (alternative to heparin)

- Dose: IV bolus of 0.1 mg/kg and an infusion of 0.25 mg/kg per hour before angiography.
- After PCI is done, an additional 0.5 mg/kg bolus is given and the infusion rate is increased to 1.75 mg/kg per hour.

LMWH (Low molecular weight heparin)

LMWH is used in non-PCI patients/late PCI (after 48 hours)

- Enoxaparin/fondaparinux
- The dose of anticoagulation drugs is the same as in STEMI

Pain relief

Pain relief is with nitrates/opioids—refer to MI chapter

Beta blockers are indicated in all patients

Metoprolol 12.5 mg bd up to 50 mg bd

Statins: As in STEMI

Complications are managed as in STEMI

- Hypoxia with oxygen target of 92%
- Cardiac failure with diuretics, ACE inhibitors, beta blockers and dobutamine

- Anticoagulation for AF + NSTEMI
- If anticoagulation is needed for patients with NSTEMI, DAPT + NOACs can be used from 1 week to 1 month depending on the bleeding and ischemic risk.
- After that, clopidogrel 75 mg od/aspirin 75 mg od and NOAC can be continued for up to 12 months if needed.
- After this, the NOAC alone can be continued.

Chapter

5

ST-Elevation Myocardial Infarction (STEMI)

Management of ST-Elevation Myocardial Infarction (STEMI)

STEMI is a medical emergency characterised by necrosis of cardiac myocytes due to compromised coronary blood supply.

Clinical Diagnosis

- Severe central chest pain is characteristic (may be absent in elderly/diabetics due to autonomic neuropathy)
- Sudden onset dyspnea
- Syncope/collapse

EMERGENCY CARE

1. Initial diagnosis
2. Relief of ischemic pain and anxiety
3. Assessment of hemodynamic state and correction of abnormalities
4. Reperfusion therapy—PCI or fibrinolysis
5. Drugs to improve long–term prognosis

INITIAL DIAGNOSIS

Comprises ECG, biomarkers, ECHO and angiography

1. ECG is the most important investigation to make an initial diagnosis

1. At least two contiguous leads with:
   a. ST-segment elevation ≥2.5 mm in men <40 years,
   b. ≥2 mm in men > 40 years,
   c. >1.5 mm in women in leads V_2–V_3 and/or
   d. 1 mm in the other leads [in the absence of left ventricular (LV) hypertrophy or left bundle branch block (LBBB)
2. Anterior wall MI-ST elevation in V_1–V_6.
3. If AVR shows >1 mm ST elevation—suggests left main block
4. In cases of inferior MI—record right precordial leads V_3R and V_4R to rule out RVMI (right ventricular MI)

5. If ST segment depression (especially with upright T-waves) is noted in V_1–V_3, record V_7–V_9 to identify posterior wall MI
6. In extensive anterior wall MI, reciprocal changes with ST depressions, may be seen in inferior leads.

Walls, ECG changes, and arteries involved

Anterior wall MI	• ST elevation V_2–V_4 • ST elevation V_1 >2.5 mm • AVR >1 mm • II, III, aVF ST depression >2 mmm • I, aVL and V_5, V_6 may have ST elevation (extensive anterior wall MI) • qRBBB pattern	Proximal LAD	Needs urgent intervention
	Diffuse ST depression with ST elevation in aVR > V_1	LMCA	
Inferior wall MI	St elevation in II, III, AVF	90% RCA 10% LCX	Look for transient complete heart block
	Lead III >II	RCA	
	St elevation II > III St elevation in V_5 and V_6, I and aVL V_1–V_3 ST depression	Left circumflex	
Right ventricular infarction (often associated with inferior wall MI)	Findings of infr wall MI+ V_1 ST elevation >1 mm and ST depression in V_2 (very specific) V_4R ST elevation	Proximal RCA	Take right leads V_3R–V_6R V_4R ST >1 mm specific watch for hypotension
Posterior wall MI (associated with lateral/inferior Wall MI)	Tall R in V_1 with R/S >1 ST depression in V_1–V_3 Tall T in same leads	Left circumflex	Record V_7–V_9 for ST elevation

7. The evolution of ST–T changes over time is depicted in Fig. 5.1.

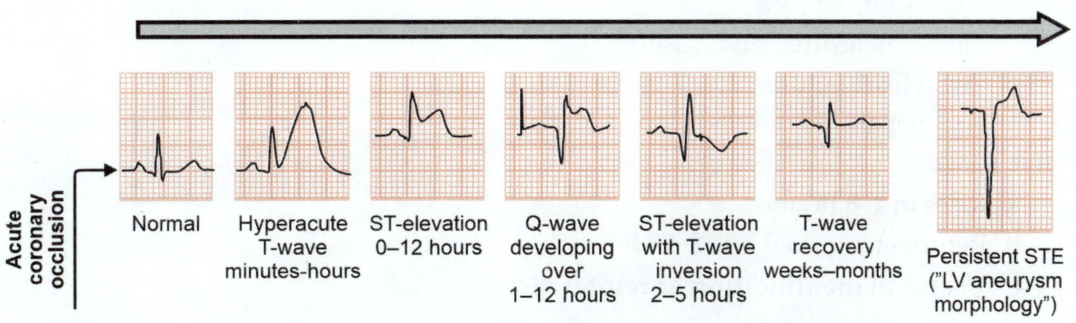

Fig. 5.1

Fallacies of ECG

- Maybe normal in the initial hours of MI. Should be repeated 1–2 hours initially, for 24 hours, if there is a strong suspicion of MI clinically.
- May be normal at the time of pain in Wellens syndrome as described below.

Wellens syndrome

Highly specific for critical stenosis of proximal LAD.

Typical features are:

- ***No ECG changes at time of pain***
- Little or no biomarker elevation
- There is no R wave loss
- Usually no ST elevation. T wave changes predominate
- Needs immediate intervention. It is of two types **(Fig. 5.2)**

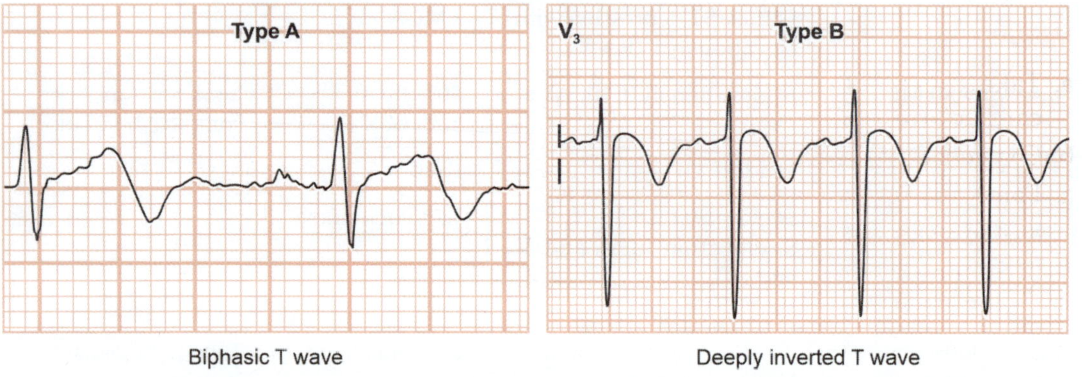

Fig. 5.1: Wellen's syndrome: Type A and Type B

2. Biomarkers: Myocardial Enzymes

i. Troponin I and T—highly sensitive, troponin T is the most reliable biomarker
   a. Both tests are positive by 4–6 hours after MI
   b. Remain elevated up to 7–10 days
   c. Should not be used as sole test for diagnosis as it can be false positive in:
      i. CKD/AKI
      ii. A fib/VT/VF
      iii. Pericarditis/myocarditis
      iv. Heart failure
      v. Sepsis

ii. CK-MB
   a. Rises in 4–8 hours
   b. Returns to normal by 48–72 hours
   c. **Useful in identification of reinfarction**
      - Myoglobin, LDH are no more used for diagnosis of MI.

3. Echo: To look for

a. LV failure (ejection fraction)
b. Regional wall motion abnormalities
c. LV aneurysm/clot
d. LV or septal rupture/free wall rupture/papillary muscle rupture
e. MR/AR/other concomitant valvular lesions

4. Coronary Angiography

Coronary angiography is done for diagnosis of culprit artery and for therapeutic intervention.

Creatinine should be normal before angiogram, as it may lead to contrast induced nephropathy if renal function is compromised. Can give $NaHCO_3$/N-acetyl cysteine in renal dysfunction.

MANAGEMENT OF STEMI

a. Take care of ABC–responsiveness, airway, breathing, circulation, if presentation with cardiac arrest follow the algorithm mentioned
b. Oxygen: Supplemental oxygen if SpO_2 <90% (target SpO_2 approx 94–95%)
c. Pain
   a. Bedrest for at least next 12 hours
   b. Sublingual nitrate
      - 5 mg dose, can be repeated for three times
      - Use IV NTG if persistent chest pain (even after 3 doses of sublingual nitrate)
      - IV nitrates should be started at 10 μg/min (= 6 mL/hr of 25 mg GTN in 250 mL dextrose and titrated every 5 minutes according to symptoms and BP.
      - Avoid nitrates in case of hypotension and RVMI
   c. Fentanyl—better side effect profile than morphine
      50–100 ug IV in 100 mL NS
   d. Inj morphine 5–10 mg IV + an antiemetic (metoclopramide 10 mg or Inj. ondansetron 4–8 mg): Watch for bradycardia while using morphine—use atropine 0.5 mg IV if it develops
   e. Inj. paracetamol 1 gm IV can also be given.

REPERFUSION THERAPY

This changes prognosis in MI, and maybe life saving in patients with large infarctions .

Types of Reperfusion Strategy

1. Percutaneous coronary intervention (PCI)
2. Fibrinolysis

Percutaneous Coronary Intervention (PCI)

- It is the preferred strategy for opening up the infarct related artery (primary PCI) in any patient presenting within 12 hours of chest pain
- Aim should be to do PCI in all patients as early as possible, with a door to needle time of 120 minutes.

- Can be done in patients presenting within 12 hours of chest pain
- Can also be done, if fibrinolysis fails/contraindications to fibrinolysis
- Also done after successful fibrinolysis within 24 hours

Fibrinolysis

It is only the second best option, and can be used to gain time if PCI capable centre is not available within 2 hours.

Contraindications to fibrinolysis:

a. Cardiogenic shock or acute severe heart failure
b. Late presentation (presented to hospital after >12 hours of onset of chest pain)
c. Electrical instability

Transfer for primary PCI is if any of these conditions (a, b, c) are present, even if the delay to revascularization will be greater than 2 hours

PRIMARY PCI STRATEGY

IRA (infarct related artery) technique

1. Stenting is recommended over balloon angioplasty
2. Stenting with DES (drug eluting stent) over BMS (bare metal stent)
3. Radial access preferred over femoral access

Periprocedural and postprocedural antithrombotic therapy for patients undergoing PCI
1. Antiplatelets
2. Anticoagulation

Doses of antiplatelets [dual antiplatelets (DAPT) needed]

Aspirin is always included
- Loading dose of 325 mg
- Followed by oral 75 mg once a day (if combined with ticagrelor)
- 150 mg/day (if combined with clopidogrel)

Second antiplatelet:
- Clopidogrel: Loading dose of 300 mg, followed by 75 mg once a day
- Ticagrelor: Loading dose of 180 mg, followed by 90 mg twice a day
- Prasugrel 60 mg loading dose, followed by 10 mg od

FIBRINOLYSIS STRATEGY

Fibrinolysis is successful when chest pain disappears and ST segment elevation resolves by 50% in 60–90 minutes. Options are:

- **tPA (alteplase)—100 mg IV over 2 hours**
  - Repeated after 15 minutes in the absence of return of spontaneous circulation (ROSC).
- Tenecteplase: Single IV bolus
  - <60 kg—30 mg (6000 IU)
  - 60–70 kg—35 mg (7000 IU)
  - 70–80 kg—40 mg (8000 IU)

- 80–90 kg—45 mg (9000 IU)
- >90 kg—50mg (10,000 IU)
- >75 years of age-reduce to half dose
- Reteplase
  - 10 units IV bolus (over 2 min), then
  - Second dose given 30 minutes after first (for total cumulative dose of 20 units)
  - In a dedicated line
- Streptokinase
  - 1.5 million units over 60 mins
  - Can cause anaphylaxis.
  - Hence steroids and chlorpheniramine can be given 30 minutes before injection. Bleeding risk is also high.
- Urokinase: 4400 units/kg IV over 10 mins followed by 4400 units/kg/hour for 12 hours.

Contraindications to fibrinolysis

Absolute contraindications

1. Prior intracranial hemorrhage/intracranial neoplasm
2. Ischemic stroke within 3 months
3. Active bleeding or bleeding diathesis (excluding menses)
4. Significant head/face trauma within 3 months

Relative contraindications

1. Severe uncontrolled hypertension (systolic >180, diastolic >110)
2. Pregnancy
3. Active peptic ulcer
4. Age >75 years
5. Current use of anticoagulant with INR >1.7 or PT (prothrombin time) >15 seconds
6. Major surgery less than 3 weeks

Interventions following fibrinolysis

a. Rescue PCI immediately when fibrinolysis has failed, i.e. < 50% reduction ST segment resolution at 60–90 mins at any time in the presence of hemodynamic or electrical instability or worsening ischemia.

b. Emergency angiography and PCI in the case of recurrent ischemia or evidence of re-occlusion after initial successful fibrinolysis.

Anticoagulation

Not needed in PCI unless there is a delay

a. Unfractionated heparin (UFH): For patients undergoing PCI—initial intravenous bolus of 70 to 100 units/kg followed by 18 units/kg infusion with target APTT of 2.5 times normal, or 5000 units SC 6th hourly

b. Low molecular weight heparin: For patients undergoing thrombolysis

- Enoxaparin IV 1 mg/kg SC every 12 hours.
- Adjustment for renal impairment/age: For patients with a creatinine clearance <30 mL/minute or >75 years of age, 1 mg/kg subcutaneously every 24 hours.

- Fondaparinux –2.5 mg SC od
- Duration: Up to 8 days (minimum of 48 hours with fibrinolysis) or until revascularization. Effective for residual thrombus

Note: Fondaparinux—not preferred in patients undergoing primary, PCI—can cause catheter thrombosis.

GP IIb/IIIa Inhibitor

Tirofiban

- Loading dose: 25 μg/kg administered over ≤5 minutes after coronary angiography, before PCI;
- Maintenance infusion: 0.15 μg/kg/min continued for up to 18 hours

Eptifibatide

- Loading dose of 180 μg/kg (maximum: 22.6 mg) over 1–2 minutes
- Followed by a continuous infusion of 2 μg/kg/min (maximum: 15 mg/hour), continued for 18 to 24 hours.

A second 180 μg/kg bolus should be given 10 minutes after the first bolus

MEDICAL MANAGEMENT

1. Maintenance Antithrombotic Strategy after STEMI

DAPT for 1 year, followed by aspirin 75 mg/day lifelong

- *For PCI:* Aspirin + ticagrelor (90 mg bd)/prasugrel (10 mg/day) (consider clopidogrel (75 mg/day) if either of these contraindicated) for 12 months after PCI
- *Fibrinolysis:* Aspirin 75 mg + clopidogrel (75 mg od)
- PPI in combination with DAPT (as high risk of GI bleed)
- If LV thrombus present, anticoagulation up to 6 months guided by repeat imaging

2. Beta Blockers—start Early

a. **Oral drugs** are indicated in cases of HF or LVEF ≤40%

b. Consider **IV beta blockers for patients undergoing PCI** (if no signs of acute HF, and with a SBP >120 mm Hg)

c. Oral metoprolol 12.5–50 mg bd

d. Routine **oral beta blockers in all cases** should be considered if not contraindicated

e. Metoprolol, carvedilol and bisoprolol are preferred.

3. Lipid Lowering Therapy

a. Obtain lipid profile in all STEMI cases

b. Tab atorvastatin 40–80 mg stat followed by high intensity statin, i.e. atorvastatin 40 mg or rosuvastatin 20–40 mg per day

c. An LDL-C goal of <70 mg/dL or at least 50% reduction should be the target.

d. In patients with recurrent events, target LDL is <55 mg/dL

4. If patient has LV dysfunction with EF < 40%, start as soon as hemodynamically stable,

ACEI/ARBs

a. Tab **ramipril** 2.5 mg per day (escalate till 20 mg per day) as single dose or two divided doses.

b. Tab **telmisartan** 40 mg od/losartan 50 mg bd/valsartan 20–80 mg/day

MRAs (mineralocorticoid receptor antagonists)—if already on ACE/ARB + beta blocker

Tab **spironolactone** 12.5–25 mg od

Tab eplerenone 25 mg od, increased over weeks to maximum of 100 mg/day

Rule out renal failure and hyperkalemia before initiation of all the above drugs.

DOSES OF MANAGEMENT OF HYPERGLYCEMIA

1. Measure glycemic status at initial evaluation in all patients.
2. If patient is on metformin and/or SGLT2 inhibitors, renal function should be carefully monitored for at least next 3 days after coronary angiography/PCI
3. Consider glucose lowering therapy in ACS if glucose >180 mg/dL
4. Use regular insulin during interventions and target blood sugar of 140–180 mg.

MANAGEMENT OF LV DYSFUNCTION, HEART FAILURE AND CARDIOGENIC SHOCK IN STEMI

1. Immediate PCI if coronary anatomy is suitable (if not suitable or PCI has failed emergency CABG is recommended)
2. Invasive BP monitoring with arterial line
3. Immediate ECHO to assess ventricular and valvular functions, detect mechanical complications
4. Can use ECMO/IABP (Impella) as support devices
5. If RV MI with cardiogenic shock—Fluids/pressors and dobutamine can be used
6. For management of cardiogenic shock (refer to Chapter 2)

MANAGEMENT OF ATRIAL FIBRILLATION

1. Acute rate control of AF

	Acute heart failure	Hypotension	Drug to be used
Scenario 1	–	–	IV beta blockers
Scenario 2	+	–	IV amiodarone
Scenario 3	+	+	IV digitalis

For AF which persists:

- If anticoagulation is needed for patients with STEMI, DAPT+ NOACs can be used from 1 week to 1 month depending on the bleeding and ischemic risk.
- After that, clopidogrel + NOAC can be continued for up to 12 months if needed. After this, the NOAC alone can be continued.

2. Cardioversion

a. Immediate electrical cardioversion is done if
   i. Adequate rate control cannot be achieved promptly with drugs in patients with AF and ongoing ischemia
   ii. Severe hemodynamic compromise
   iii. Heart failure

b. IV amiodarone after electrical cardioversion in unstable patient with recent onset AF.

MANAGEMENT OF VENTRICULAR ARRHYTHMIAS AND CONDUCTION DISTURBANCES IN THE ACUTE PHASE

1. IV beta blockers for polymorphic VT (lignocaine may work) and/or VF /VPCs
2. IV amiodarone, if recurrent polymorphic VT
3. Correct electrolytes: Keep K >4 mEq/L, and Mg >2 mEq/L
4. In cases of hemodynamic instability with high degree AV block without stable escape rhythm
   a. IV positive chronotropic meds-epinephrine/vasopressin/atropine
   b. Temporary pacing in inferior wall MI (usually transient blocks). In anterior wall MI-may need permanent pacing rarely.
   c. Consider for intracardiac defibrillator if EF is <35% after 40 days
   d. Urgent angiography with a view to revascularization is indicated if patient has not received previous reperfusion therapy

Chapter

6

Supraventricular Tachycardia (SVT)

Definition of tachycardia—heart rate of more than 100 bpm.

Classification of tachycardias (based on the QRS complex)

1. Narrow QRS complex (<120 ms)
   a. Regular (supraventricular tachycardia: SVT)
      i. Atrioventricular re-entry tachycardia (AVRT)
      ii. Atrioventricular nodal re-entry tachycardia (AVNRT)
   b. Irregular
      i. Atrial fibrillation (refer to Chapter 8: Atrial Fibrillation)
      ii. Atrial tachycardia/flutter with varying conduction block
      iii. Multifocal atrial tachycardia
2. Wide QRS complex (>120 msecs)
   Regular:
   - Ventricular tachycardia (refer to Chapter 7: Ventricular Tachycardia)
   - SVT with aberrancy

   Irregular
   - Af with aberrancy
   - Polymorphic VT
   - Torsades de pointes

Clinical features of supraventricular tachycardia

- Palpitations: Sudden onset, sudden offset
- Syncope: If ventricular rate is high
- Chest pain: If underlying IHD
- **Hypotension:** This decides the management
- Worsening of heart failure symptoms

Investigations

- Investigations: ECG to identify type of tachycardia
- Holter monitoring may be needed to diagnose paroxysmal tachycardia

ECHO: To rule out structural heart disease

ECG OF SVT

- **AVNRT—Atrioventricular node reentry tachycardia**
  - *Functional* reentry circuit within the AV node
  - Regular tachycardia ~140–280 bpm.
  - QRS narrow (<120 ms) unless pre-existing bundle branch block, accessory pathway, or rate related aberrant conduction.
  - P wave, if visible exhibit *retrograde conduction* with inversion in leads II, III, aVF.

    P may be buried in the QRS complex, or visible after/before (rarely) the QRS complex.
  - RP interval shorter than 70 ms.
  - Pseudo S in lead III, pseudo R in V1.

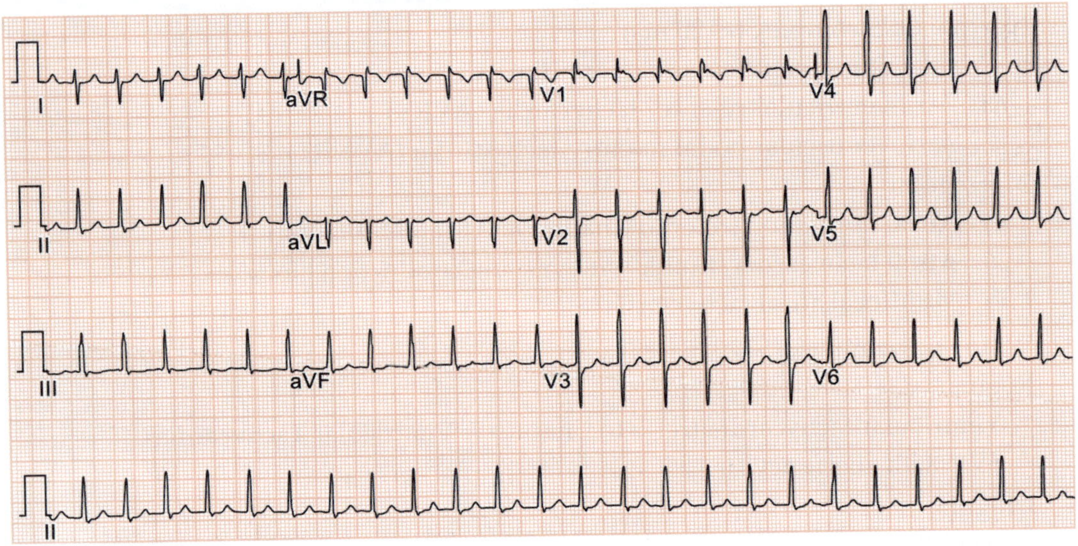

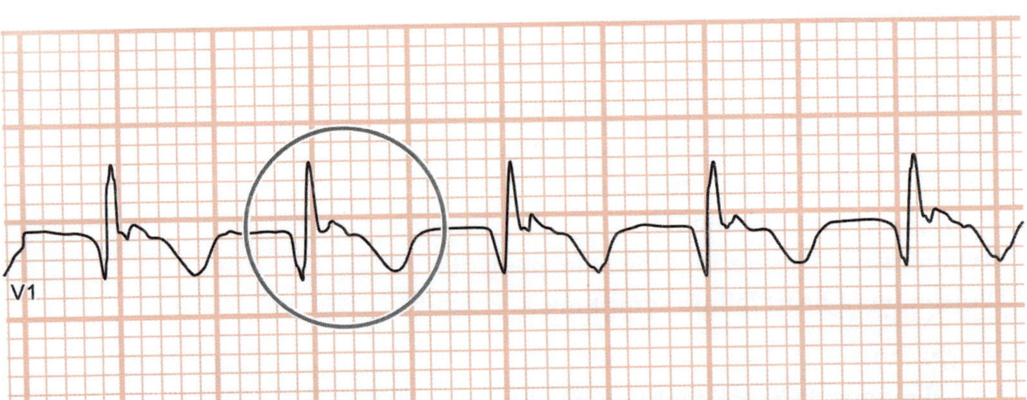

Fig. 6.1: Narrow complex tachycardia P wave after R wave in rhythm strip

a. AVRT—Atrioventricular reentry tachycardia (WPW syndrome)

- Early activation of the ventricles: Impulses bypassing the AV node through an accessory pathway. Through the Bundle of Kent it is called Wolff-Parkinson-White syndrome (WPW)
- PR interval <120 ms
- Delta wave—slurring/slow rise of initial portion of the QRS
- QRS prolongation >110 ms
- ST segment and T wave discordant changes, and QRS alternans
- V1 is positive in left accessory pathway, negative V1 is right accessory pathway
- Pseudo-infarction pattern: 70% of patients – due to negatively deflected delta waves in the inferior/anterior leads ("pseudo-Q waves"), or as a prominent R wave in V1–3 (mimicking posterior infarction).
- RP interval longer than 70 ms.

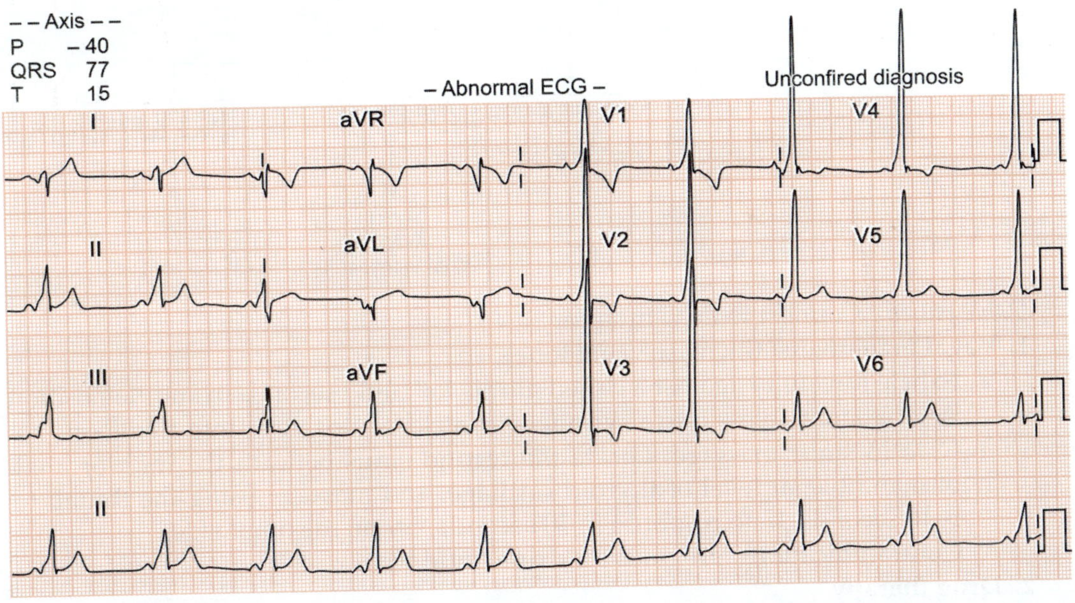

Management of SVT

- *Unstable patient* (patient with hypotension):

  Synchronized cardioversion:
  - Narrow regular—100 to 200 J
  - Narrow irregular—100 to 200 J
  - Wide regular—200 J
  - Wide irregular—200 J defibrillation dose to be given

Flowchart 6.1: Approach to ECG diagnosis narrow complex tachycardia

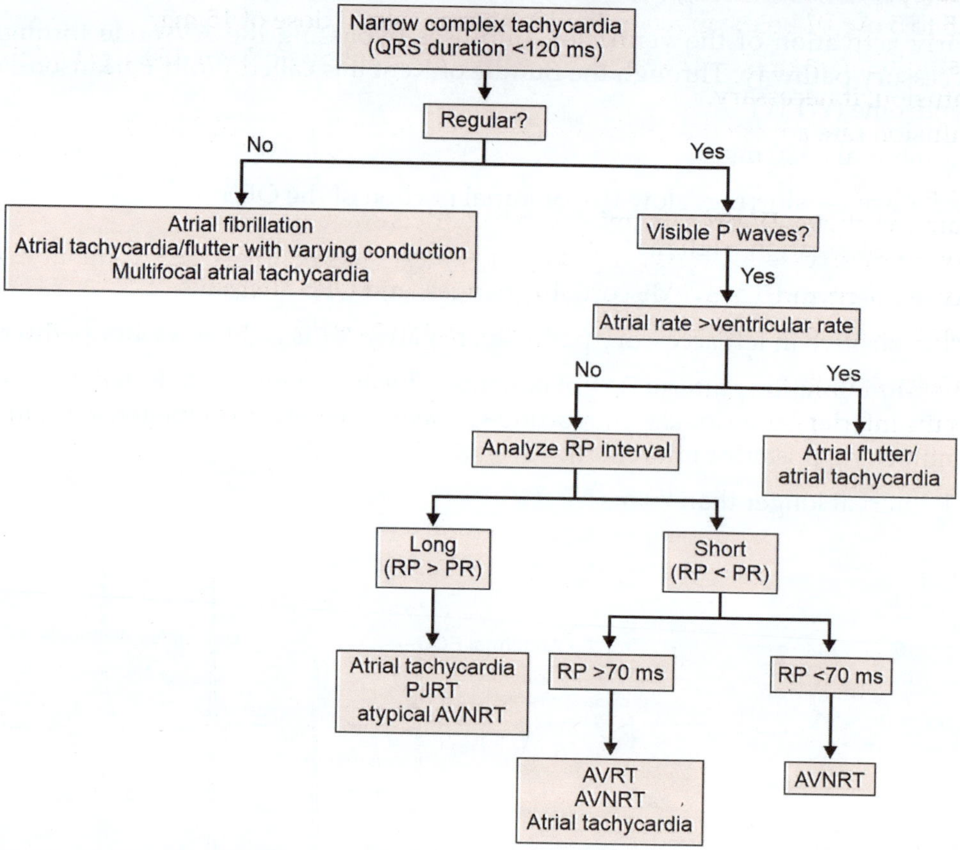

- *Stable patient:* Connect to ECG monitor
  1. **Vagal maneuvers** (increase vagal tone)
     a. Exhale forcefully against a closed glottis for 10–15 seconds in supine position; Ask patient to blow into a syringe with a closed nozzle or into a balloon
     b. Carotid sinus massage: Locate the carotid sinus beneath the inferior angle of mandible, at level of thyroid cartilage, and massage using the thumb for 5–10 seconds. If no response in 30 seconds, try on the other side. Contraindications: previous TIA, or carotid bruit
  2. **Drug therapy**
     - **Adenosine**
       - First dose: 6 mg rapid IV push followed by saline flush.
       - Second dose: 12 mg if required (persisting SVT after 3 minutes from first dose); (max total dose—18 mg)
       - Avoid in severe IHD or bronchial asthma
- **Verapamil:** 5 to 10 mg IV bolus over 2 minutes;
  If no response, an additional 10 mg IV bolus given 15 to 30 minutes following the initial dose.
- **Diltiazem:** 0.25 mg/kg (average dose 20 mg) IV bolus over 2 minutes; If no response, an additional 0.35 mg/kg (average dose 25 mg) IV bolus may be administered 15 to 30 minutes following the initial dose.

- **Metoprolol:** 2.5 to 5 mg IV bolus over 2 to 5 minutes; If no response, an additional 2.5 to 5 mg IV bolus given every 10 minutes—total dose of 15 mg.
- **Esmolol:** 1 mg/kg IV bolus over 30 seconds, followed by a 150 μg/kg/minute infusion, if necessary.
  Infusion rate adjusted to maintain desired heart rate (up to 300 μg/kg/minute).

WPW Syndrome

- Same as above: IV procainamide can be added if refractory
- Avoid digoxin even in AF, as it may increase ventricular rate
- Avoid adenosine and other AV blocking agents like digoxin
- Radiofrequency ablation—refer to electrophysiologist.

Catheter Ablation

If recurrent, dangerous and refractory to therapy. Refer to an electrophysiologist.

Chapter

7

Ventricular Tachycardia (VT)

Ventricular arrhythmia includes ventricular tachycardia (VT) and ventricular fibrillation (VF). For VF, refer to Chapter 1: Cardiac Arrest.

Common presenting symptoms are

- Palpitations
- Syncope
- Sudden cardiac death/cardiac arrest
- Rarely asymptomatic—in normal hearts

VT is Classified as

1. **Non-sustained VT**

   3 or more consecutive ventricular complexes (rate 100/min) that terminate within 30 seconds.
2. **Sustained monomorphic VT (similar morphology)**

   >3 ventricular ectopics, monomorphic, lasts >30 seconds, or causes hemodynamic collapse
   - Polymorphic VT
     - 3 or more ventricular complexes varying in morphology lasts >30 seconds.
     - Torsades de pointes, is one variety with prolonged QT interval (>460 ms in men or >480 ms in women)

A. **Monomorphic ventricular tachycardia**

Most common causes are:

- Structural heart disease—ischemic heart disease
- Dilated cardiomyopathy
- HOCM
- Postcardiac surgery scars

ECG features

- Rate of >100 bpm;
- Broad QRS complex >120 ms, usually >160 ms
- ***Extreme axis deviation*** ('northwest axis')—QRS positive in aVR and negative in I and aVF.
- ***AV dissociation*** (P and QRS complexes at different rates).

- ***Capture beats***—sinoatrial node transiently 'captures' the ventricles, QRS complex of normal duration.
- ***Fusion beats***—occur when a sinus and ventricular beat coincide to produce a hybrid complex of intermediate morphology.
- ***Positive or negative concordance***, i.e. leads V_1–V_6 show entirely positive (R) or entirely negative (QS) complexes, with no RS complexes seen.
- RSR′ complexes with a taller "left rabbit ear". This is the most specific finding in favor of VT. This is in contrast to RBBB, where the right rabbit ear is taller.

Brugada criteria to differentiate between VT and SVT

If the answer to any of these is yes, it is VT.
- Absence of RS complex in any lead
- RS complex in any lead with RS interval >100 ms
- AV dissociation
- Morphological criteria present for VT present from V_1 to V_6

B. **Polymorphic VT and torsades de pointes**

Torsades de pointes (TdP) is a specific form of PVT with QT prolongation; Characteristic morphology: QRS complexes "twist" around the isoelectric line, as shown in **Fig. 7.1**.

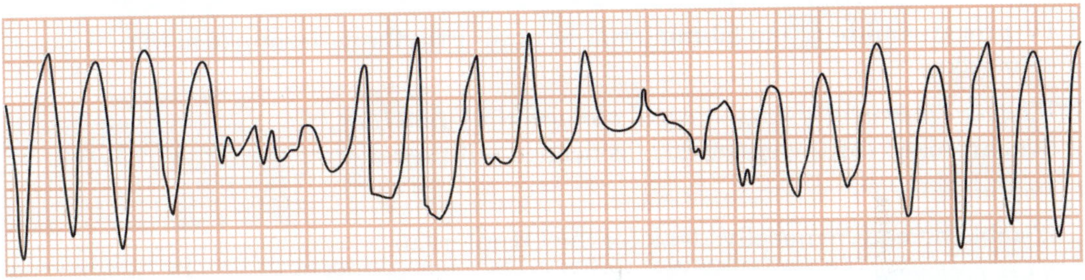

Fig. 7.1: Torsades de pointes

Due to multiple ventricular foci resulting in QRS complexes varying in amplitude, axis and duration.

Causes

- **Commonest cause of PVT is myocardial ischemia/infarction.**
- Electrolyte imbalance (QT prolongation): Hypokalemia and hyperkalemia, hypomagnesemia, hypocalcemia
- Hypoxia and acidosis
- Drugs (QT prolongation): Antipsychotics, tricyclic antidepressants, amiodarone, chloroquine, azithromycin and fluoroquinolones.

Management of ventricular arrhythmias

Sustained monomorphic VT

1. ***If hemodynamically unstable:*** Common in polymorphic VT than monomorphic VT
   - Monomorphic VT: Synchronized cardioversion 200 J.
   - If polymorphic VT: Unsynchronized DC shocks 200 J, as monitor may not recognize synchronization.

If no pulse is felt, treat as pulseless VF: Start CPR simultaneously (refer to Chapter 1: Cardiac Arrest).

2. ***If hemodynamically stable and normal LV function***
   - **IV amiodarone**—contraindicated in hypotension
   - First dose—150 mg bolus over 10 minutes. Repeat if needed.
   - Followed by infusion: 1 mg/min for the first 6 hours, then 0.5 mg/min × 18 h
     - (1 vial—150 mg; 6 vials (900 mg) in 450 mL NS is 2 mg/mL—to be infused as 30 mL/hr for first 6 hours, followed by 15 mL/hr for 18 hours)

       Same dose can be given in 5% dextrose, except in diabetics.
   - PO: 400 mg q 8 to 12 h for 1–2 weeks, then 300–400 mg daily; reduce dose to 200 mg daily if possible

   IV lidocaine (1 to 1.5 mg/kg [typically 75 to 100 mg] at 25 to 50 mg/min; 0.5 to repeat 0.75 mg/kg every 5 to 10 min if needed, especially in acute MI).

   IV beta blockers
   - IV sotalol: 100 mg over 5 minutes
   - Metoprolol IV: 5 mg over 5 min up to 3 doses
   - PO: 25–100 mg extended release qd or q12h

   IV procainamide (20 to 50 mg/minute until arrhythmia terminates. Max dose of 17 mg/kg)
3. ***If hemodynamically unstable and abnormal LV function***

   Synchronized cardioversion 200 J is needed with sedation.
4. ***Polymorphic VT***

   If stable hemodynamically: look for the QT interval.

   If QT prolonged
   - Look for causes such as hypokalemia and hypomagnesemia, drug toxicity and correct
   - For torsades de pointes QT : IV magnesium sulphate 2 gm IV stat.
   - In case of recurrence: Isoproterenol infusion up to 20 µg/min to increase the heart rate >120/min

   If normal QT
   - Look for underlying cardiac disease and treat

For prevention of future arrhythmias especially in long QT syndromes: Beta blockers
- Metoprolol XR (25–100 mg bd)
- Carvedilol (3.125–25 mg bd)
- Bisoprolol (2–10 mg bd)

Amiodarone 200 mg od or bd—if QT is normal only

Device therapy/electrophysiological intervention

- ICD in all survivors of cardiac arrest with ventricular fibrillation or unstable VTs due to irreversible causes or structural heart disease
- Catheter based RFA in structurally normal hearts associated with VT.

Chapter

8

Atrial Fibrillation (AF)

It is a common form of atrial arrhythmia

Types

- Paroxysmal (resolves within 7 days)
- Persistent (>7 days),
- Permanent (>1 year or refractory to cardioversion)
- Recurrent (if two or more episodes)

Clinical Symptoms

- May be asymptomatic
- Palpitations/dyspnea/angina
- Presyncope, or infrequently, syncope

Aetiology: Common Causes

- Hypertension
- IHD
- Valvular heart disease
- Cardiomyopathy
- Pulmonary embolism
- COPD
- Alcohol
- Thyrotoxicosis
- Lone AF—no cause found

Clinical Symptoms

- Palpitations—irregular
- Syncope—if ventricular rate is fast
- Chest pain—can be precipitated if rate is fast and there is IHD underlying

Clinical Signs

- Irregularly irregular pulse
- Absent a waves in JVP
- Varying BP—take average of 3 recordings
- Varying S1. Absent S4.

AF is Associated with the Following Changes on ECG

- No discrete P waves.
- Varying R-R interval
- The QRS complexes are narrow

Calculating Ventricular Rate

The ventricular rate >100/min if there is no AV nodal delay. Count this rate by counting the number of RRs in 6 seconds. Multiply by 10.

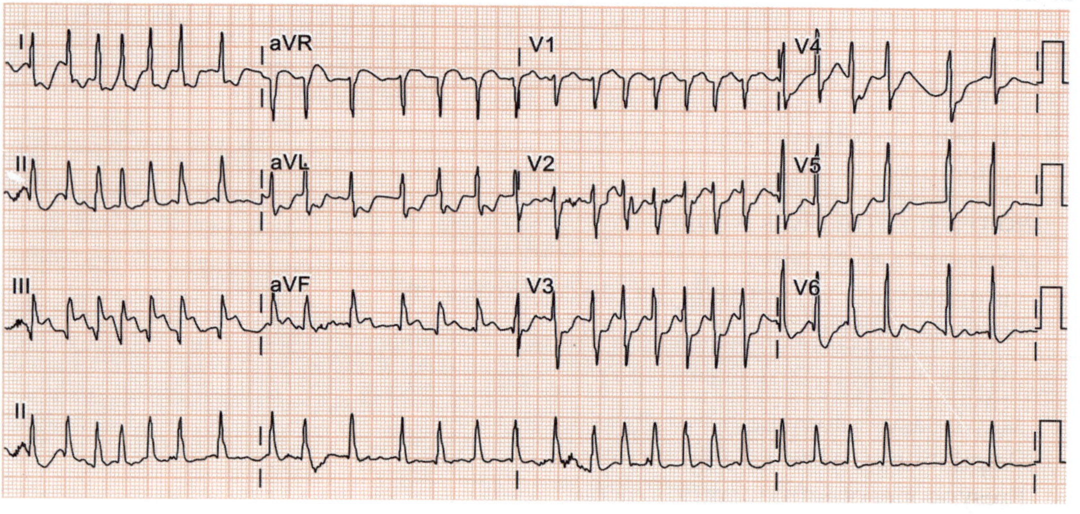

Fig. 8.1: AF with fast ventricular response

MANAGEMENT

- Atrial fibrillation causes hemodynamic compromise only if there is fast ventricular rate (FVR).
- Anticoagulation is necessary for all atrial fibrillation due to underlying valvular and structural heart disease, irrespective of ventricular rate.

The treatment of AF with fast ventricular rate (FVR), involves these decisions:

1. Choosing between rhythm control and rate control
2. Determining the urgency of initial therapy—emergent, urgent or elective
3. Decision to start anticoagulation and its timing

1. Choosing between Rate and Rhythm Control

Rate control is done, when the possibility of recurrence is high:

- Long standing AF
- Established valvular heart disease
- Large left atrium
- Advanced age
- Pulmonary/thyroid disease

Helps by decreasing ventricular rate, by increasing refractory period of AV node. This leads to better stroke volume, and decreased myocardial oxygen demand. Thus, it helps in heart failure.

Disadvantage: Risk of embolism remains.

Rhythm control helps by establishing sinus rhythm, and has the additional advantage of no embolic risk.

2. Urgency of Therapy

Emergent therapy: Rhythm control

If hemodynamically unstable: Hypotension, pulmonary edema, myocardial ischemia.

Treatment: Immediate DC cardioversion and/or pharmacological IV cardioversion

a. Electrical Cardioversion (rhythm control)

- Sedate with injection fentanyl (50–100 μg IV) or midazolam (1–2 mg IV).
- Blood pressure, heart rate, oxygen saturation monitored.
- 100–200 J DC synchronised cardioversion.
- If restoration of sinus rhythm fails, another 360 J DC cardioversion may be attempted.

Note

- There is a risk of thromboembolism when sinus rhythm is restored. However, there is no time to wait for anticoagulation in these patients, as this is a life-threatening emergency.
- Anticoagulate for 4 weeks, immediately post-DCC after restoration of sinus rhythm. Further anticoagulation to be decided based on CHA2DS2VASc score and any recurrence.
- In those who fail pharmacological cardioversion, anticoagulate for 3 weeks, do TEE, then take up for DCC.

b. Pharmacologic Cardioversion (rhythm control)

Rhythm control is preferred for long term management if

- <65 yr age
- >65 yr and symptomatic despite rate control

- **Amiodarone**
  - IV amiodarone **150 mg over 10 minutes**, followed by infusion in 5% dextrose, **1 mg/minute for six hours**, then **0.5 mg/minute for 18 hours**/change to oral maintenance dosing (e.g. 100 to 200 mg tid).
  - Drug of choice for AF + structural heart disease
- **Flecainide**
  - IV flecainide 2 mg/kg over 10 min acutely reverts AF in 6 hours.
  - An oral dose of 200 to 300 mg/single, large oral dose of flecainide (100 to 400 mg) is effective for AF reversal.
  - Always start beta blockers before flecainide, as it may otherwise increase AV conduction and cause VF.
  - C/I in cases of moderate to severe LV dysfunction.
- **Propafenone**
  - IV propafenone 2 mg/kg over 10 to 20 min
  - Oral propafenone: Large dose of 450 to 600 mg.
  - Given with food to increase bioavailability.

Ibutilide

- Ibutilide IV 1 mg over 10 minutes. Repeat once after 20 minutes, if needed.
- Patient should be monitored for next 6–8 hours (risk of ventricular arrhythmia)
- C/I if QT >440 ms
- TEE mandatory before giving drug

Note

Start anticoagulation with IV heparin or subcutaneous LMWH immediately before pharmacological cardioversion. Change to NOAC's/VKA (target INR 2–3) for 4 weeks after reversal to sinus rhythm. Further anticoagulation to be decided on CHA2DS2VASc Score and recurrence of AF.

URGENT THERAPY

- Hemodynamically stable but symptomatic.
- Not fulfilling indications for pharmacological cardioversion.

Initial treatment: **intravenous rate control as described below,** followed by oral drugs

A. Beta blockers

- **Esmolol**
  - A bolus of 0.5 mg/kg IV over 1 min, followed by infusion at 50 μg/kg per min.
  - Repeat bolus dose after every 5 minutes to a maximum of 3 doses if heart rate is not controlled.
  - Increase infusion dose by 50 μg/kg every 5 minutes after the bolus doses to a maximum of 200 μg/kg per min.
- **Propranolol**
  - IV propranolol, 1 mg over one minute. Repeat every 2–5 minutes to a total of 5 mg. Repeat after 4 hours.
- **Metoprolol**
  - IV bolus of 2.5 to 5.0 mg over 2 minutes.
  - Repeated at 5 minutes intervals up to a total of 15 mg as needed.
  - Change to oral formulation once rate is controlled.

B. Calcium Channel Blockers

- **Diltiazem**
  - IV bolus of 0.25 mg/kg (average adult dose 20 mg) over two minutes.
  - Wait for 15 minutes. If no 20% reduction in heart rate or heart rate >100 beats/min, a second bolus of 0.35 mg/kg (average adult dose 25 mg) is given over two minutes.
  - In those who respond to boluses, a continuous infusion at a rate of 5 to 15 mg/h is initiated.
  - This regimen usually controls the ventricular rate within 5 minutes.
- **Verapamil**
  - IV 5 to 10 mg over 2–3 minutes, repeated every 15 to 30 minutes.
  - Once rate control is achieved with IV bolus (often 1–2 are needed), start a maintenance infusion at a rate of 5 mg/hour

- **Contraindication to diltiazem and verapamil**
  - Severe heart failure (New York Heart Failure, class III or IV)
  - Significant hypotension
  - Preexcitation syndrome
  - Sinus node dysfunction

Note

Patient managed chronically with a rate control strategy can be taken up for cardioversion after adequate anticoagulation for 3 weeks. Continue anticoagulation thereafter for 4 weeks.

IV heparin (LMWH or unfractionated). Overlap with warfarin to target INR of 2–3 or NOACs.

Further anticoagulation to be decided based on CHA2DS2VASc score and any recurrence

ELECTIVE THERAPY

Indications

- Patients who have mild or no symptoms.
- Underlying heart disease
- Target heart rate: 70–80/min

Beta blockers, calcium channel blockers

- *Metoprolol:* 50–100 mg bd/day
- *Verapamil:* 80 mg tid. Maximum dose: 480 mg/day
- *Diltiazem:* 120–240 mg/day. Maximum dose: 540 mg/day

Flowchart 8.1: Approach to emergency/urgent therapy

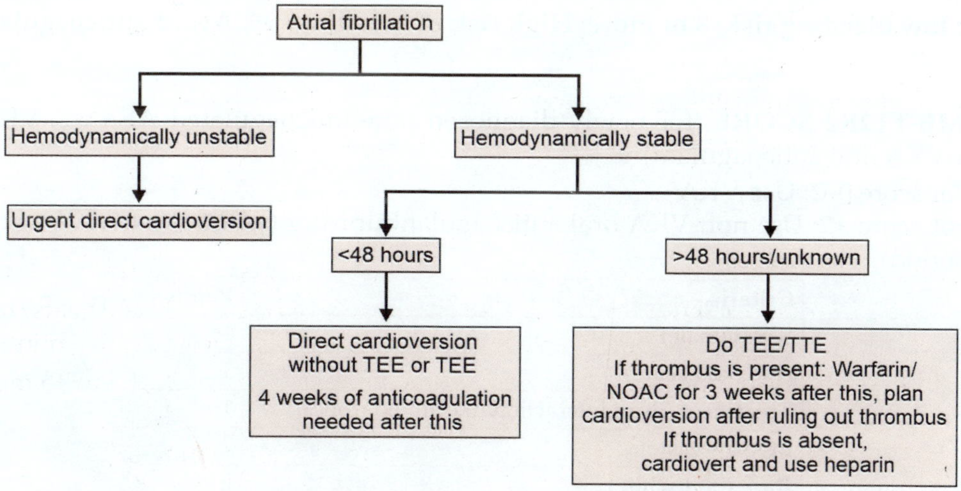

3. Anticoagulation

Needed for paroxysmal, persistent or permanent AF. Unless AF is reverted to sinus rhythm.

For rheumatic AF and valvular heart disease associated AF anticoagulation is a must, and is lifelong. VKA preferred.

In non-rheumatic AF: Check CHA2DS2VASc score:

CHA2DS2VASc risk factor points	Score
Congestive heart Failure	1
Hypertension	1
Age ≥75	2
Diabetes mellitus	1
Stroke, TIA or thromboembolism in past	2
Vascular disease (prior MI/PVD/aortic aneurysm)	1
Age 65–74 years	1
Sex category—female	1

Any score > 2 needs anticoagulation in both sexes.

HASBLED SCORE

This helps to calculate the bleeding risk. This must be balanced with benefit when anticoagulation is done.

Condition	Points
Hypertension > 160 mm systolic	1
Abnormal renal/liver function	1 for each
Stroke	1
Bleeding	1
Labile INRs	1
Elderly> 65 years	1
Drugs/ethanol	1

0–2: low bleeding risk; 3 or more: High risk of bleeding; >5: Avoid anticoagulation

Choice of Anticoagulant

SAME-TT2R2 SCORE (for newly diagnosed non-anticoagulated AF case, VKA *vs* non-VKA oral anticoagulant)

- For score 0–2: Use VKA
- For score >2: Use non-VKA oral anticoagulant upfront (without a trial of warfarin period)

Criteria	Points
Sex (female)	1
Age (<60 years)	1
Treatment (drug interaction like amiodarone)	1
Medical history*	2
Race (non-white)	2
Tobacco use (within 2 years)	2
Maximum points	8

* Any two of the following: HTN, DM, CAD, MI, PAD, CHF, previous stroke, pulmonary disease, hepatic disease or renal disease.

Intervention for AF-ablation

Indications:

- Symptomatic despite medical management
- AF related cardiomyopathy
- Young pts with paroxysmal AF

Surgical techniques:

- Maze procedure can be done.
- Left atrial appendage ligation at time of MVR/other cardiac surgeries

ATRIAL FLUTTER

- Atrial rate: 200–400/minute
- Ventricular rate depends on AV block. Usually 2:1, hence characteristic ventricular rate of 150/min. Can be 3:1, or 4:1 also. Can have varying blocks also.
- The pulse may be regular or slightly irregular
- Hypotension: If ventricular rate is very fast, but normal BP is more common

Clinical features

- Palpitations
- Syncope
- Cardiac failure
- Chest pain

ECG features: Saw toothed appearance of regular P waves as seen below in this ECG

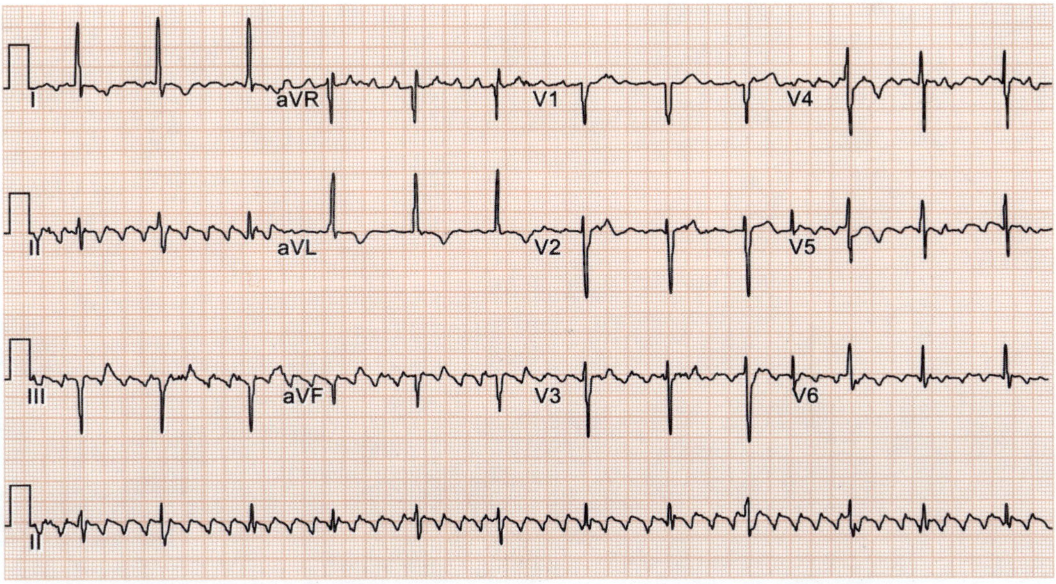

TREATMENT OF ATRIAL FLUTTER

Radiofrequency ablation: Treatment of choice, much better than medical treatment.

Medical management (same as atrial fibrillation)

- If hemodynamically unstable and <48 hours, cardioversion, as in atrial fibrillation (AF)—95% successful.
- Anticoagulation post-DC version is needed
- Pharmacological cardioversion, like in AF, is also an option.

If >48 hours, anticoagulation should be started and managed as in AF. Rate control with beta blockers, calcium channel blockers like in AF.

Chapter

9

Bradycardia

Definition: Heart rate less than 60 bpm.

Bradycardia is due to:

1. Disorders of the SA node
2. Disorders of the AV node
3. Ventricular escape rhythms—idioventricular

Disorders of the SA node

1. Sinus bradycardia
2. Sinoatrial exit block
3. Sinus pause
4. Sinus arrest (if pause >3 secs)
5. Sick sinus syndrome

Etiology of the SA node disease:

Extrinsic	Intrinsic
Autonomic • Carotid sinus hypersensitivity • Vasovagal stimulation	Acute MI – especially inferior wall MI
Drugs • Beta blockers • CCB • Digoxin • Anti-arrhythmic drugs and adenosine	Inflammatory • Pericarditis • Myocarditis when it causes bradycardia • Rheumatic heart disease
Hypothyroidism Hypoxia and sleep apnea Obstructive jaundice Increased intracranial pressure	Sick sinus syndrome Congenital heart block Post-surgical disease

Note

Extrinsic causes of SA node are usually reversible

Clinical Features

- Heart rate <60 bpm normal in young athletes. No structural heart disease and asymptomatic
- Bradycardia may cause fatigue, pre-syncope, syncope, hypotension, angina, worsening of heart failure, exercise intolerance, in abnormal hearts.

- In sinus syndrome—tachy-brady variant symptoms of tachycardia might also be present such as palpitations and angina.
- The alternating tachycardia and bradycardia also increases the risk of thrombo-embolism

Investigations

ECG: Will include sinus bradycardia, sinus pauses, sinus arrest, and sinus exit block and chronotropic incompetence. 12 lead standard ECG will show:

1. **Sinus bradycardia**
   - Sinus rhythm
   - P waves prior to every QRS complex which is positive in lead I, II and aVL and negative in aVR
   - Normal PR interval

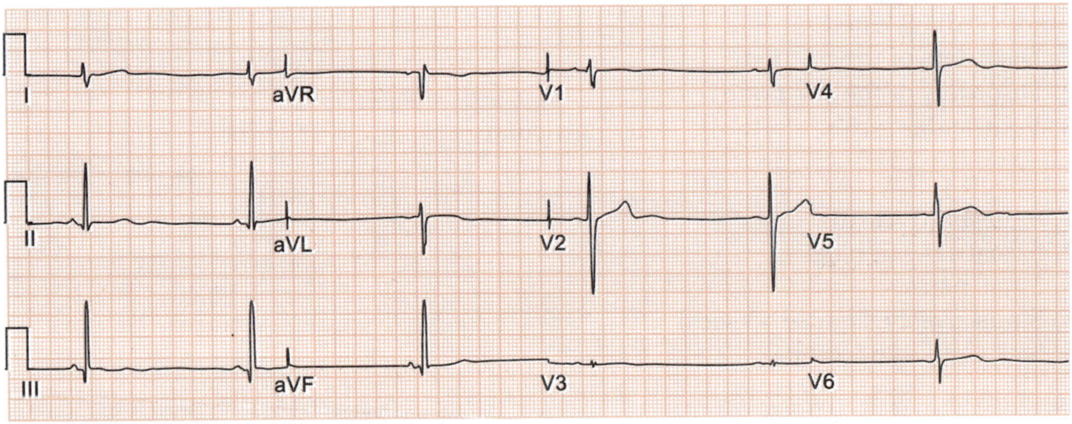

2. **Sinus arrest and sinus pause**
   - Prolonged absence of sinus node activity (absent P waves) >3 seconds
   - The P–P interval delimiting the pause does not equal a multiple of the basic P–P interval.

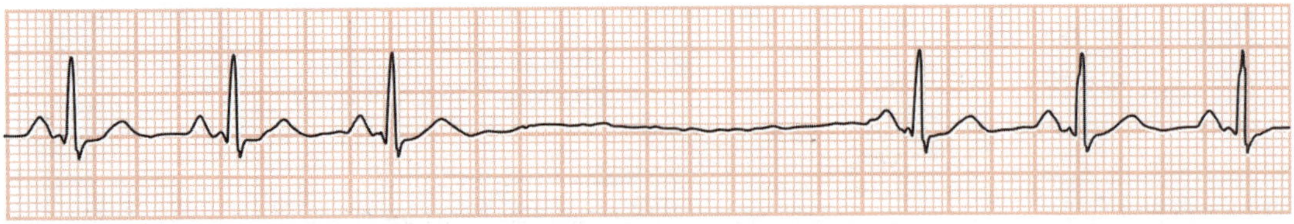

3. **Sick sinus syndrome—tachycardia bradycardia syndrome**
   - The sinus rate is extremely slow, varying from 40 bpm to around 10 bpm in places.
   - Sinus bradycardia alternating with supraventricular tachycardia (most commonly A fib).

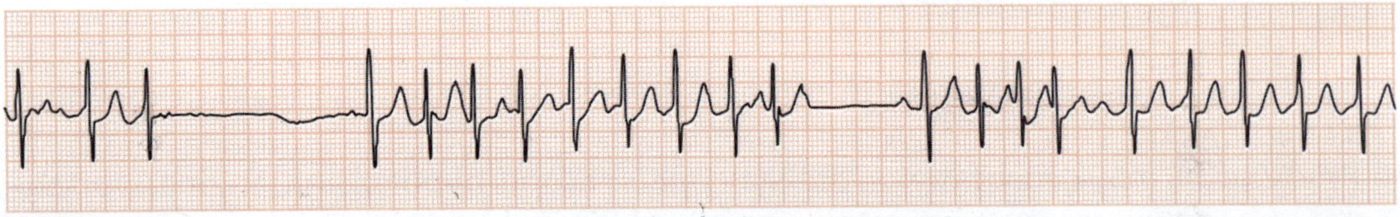

Treatment

- If asymptomatic—no treatment is required
- If patient is hemodynamically unstable then:
  - Inj atropine 0.5 mL IV stat and can be repeated every 3 to 5 minutes. Maximum of 3 mg.
  - If there is no improvement with atropine, temporary cardiac pacing should be considered.
  - Dopamine and epinephrine can also be considered if cardiac pacing is not available
- If the patient is symptomatic but hemodynamically stable
  - Treat cause
  - For MI-revascularization
  - For drug-withdraw
  - The underlying cause for the bradycardia should be identified and corrected. For example, in case of MI causing bradycardia, immediate coronary revascularization should be attempted. In case of drug induced bradycardia, the suspect drug should be withdrawn.

Disorders of the AV node

Bradycardia can be caused by delay in conduction of impulses from atria to ventricle–causing varying degree of heart block.

Can be transient/permanent. Functional or anatomical.

First degree block:

Delayed conduction from the atrium to the ventricle (defined as a prolonged PR interval of >200 milliseconds or corrected for heart rate) without interruption in atrial to ventricular conduction.

- Site of delay can include atria, AV node, bundle of His, or Purkinje fibres.
- Usually does not cause hemodynamic instability and is found incidentally on ECGs.
- Does not require treatment.

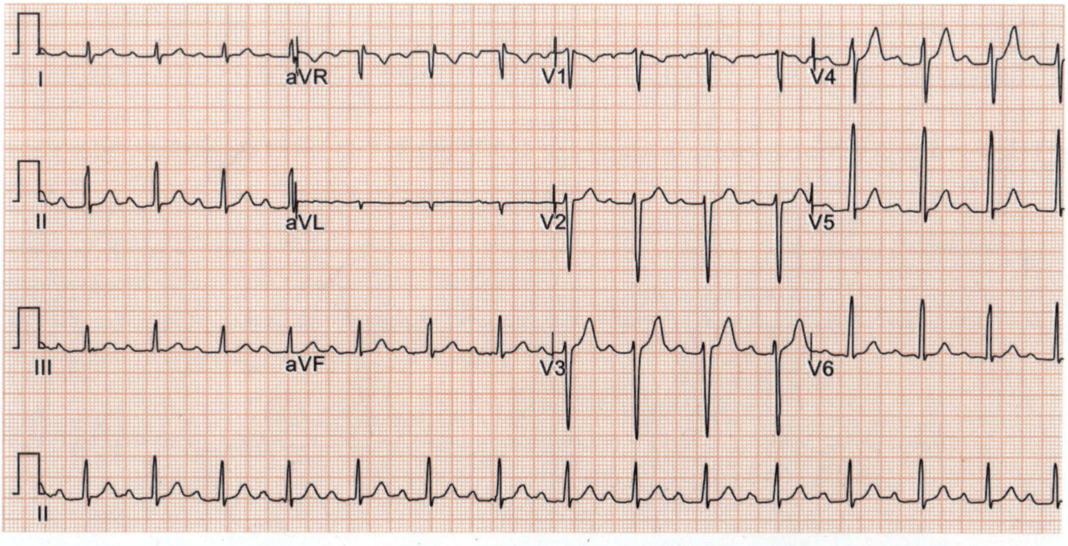

Second degree heart block

- Further classified into:
    - Mobitz type I (Wenckebach)—progressive lengthening of PR interval followed by dropped beat non-conduction
    - Mobitz type II second degree AV block—occasional/repetitive sudden block of conduction
- Mobitz type II has a poorer prognosis. It usually presents with hemodynamic instability. It also has a greater risk of proceeding to complete heart block.

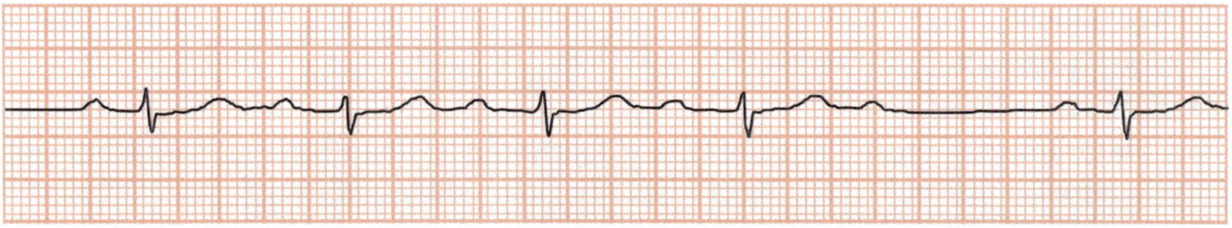

Mobitz Type I

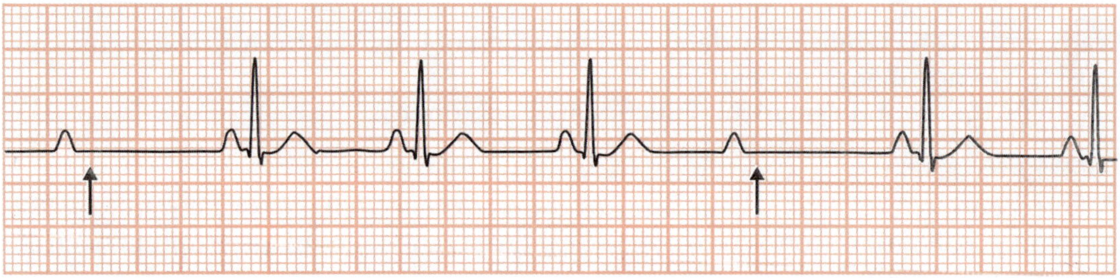

Mobitz Type II

Complete heart block:

- No atrial impulses conduct to the ventricle.
- The rhythm is maintained by a junctional or ventricular escape rhythm.
- The patient may suffer ventricular stand still leading to syncope (if self-terminating) or sudden cardiac death (if prolonged).
- High-grade AV block—Infra-hisian type II AV block and third degree AV blocks

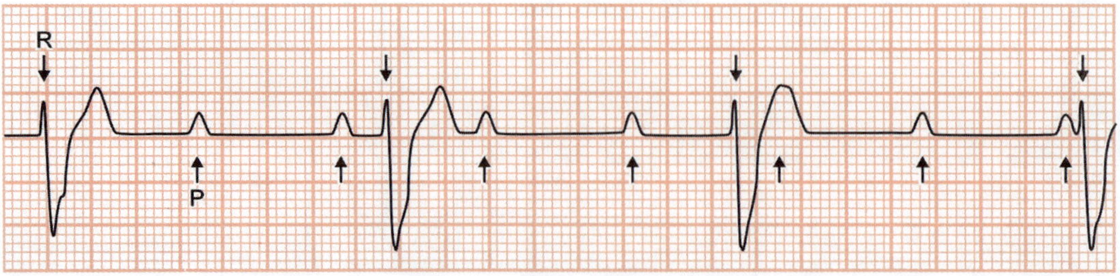

Management

- Reversible causes of bradycardia should be identified and corrected
- If no reversible cause is found then a permanent pacemaker should be inserted
- Indications of pacing
    - Persistent bradycardia
        - Sinus node disease (symptoms present and attributable to bradycardia)
        - Acquired AV block (irrespective of symptoms)
            - Third degree
            - Second degree type 2 AV block
    - Intermittent bradycardia
        - Sinus node disease—documentation of symptomatic bradycardia due to sinus arrest or sinus-atrial block
        - Intermittent/paroxysmal AV block—third degree or second degree
- Transcutaneous pacing—only for a brief amount of time.
- Central venous access—for urgent transvenous pacing.

Drug Therapy

Initial dose of atropine is 0.6 mg, can be repeated after 3–5 mins to a total dose of 3 mg.

- IV and/or oral theophylline (150 mg bd), can be used both for acute and chronic bradycardia, as a temporary measure only. Care should be taken in patients with a structural heart disease.
- Orciprenaline 10 mg tid, for sinus bradycardia/complete heart block.
- IV dopamine (2–5 μg/kg/min) and dobutamine (3–5 μg/kg/min) infusions can be used for patients with heart failure with bradycardia.
- Epinephrine infusion can also be considered.

Chapter

10

Cardiac Tamponade

Cardiac tamponade refers to the accumulation of pericardial fluid, blood, or pus in pericardial space, leading to an increase in intrapericardial pressure, thereby reducing ventricular filling and decreasing cardiac output.

Etiology

- Malignancy (breast, lung, thyroid cancer, and lymphoma)
- Uremia
- Ventricular free wall rupture following MI
- Dressler's syndrome
- Penetrating trauma
- Tuberculosis

- Less common causes:
  - Radiation
  - Myxedema
  - Systemic lupus erythematosus (SLE)
  - Infection: Viral, bacterial

Classification

- Acute cardiac tamponade: Within minutes
- Subacute/chronic cardiac tamponade: Days to weeks

Clinical Features

- The rapidity of fluid collection, rather than the amount of fluid, has a greater impact on the severity of clinical signs and symptoms.
- Dyspnea
- Chest pain: Substernal chest discomfort, radiating to neck and jaw, exacerbated by inspiration, and improved with sitting forward
- Fever, if infection
- Abdominal discomfort or nausea: Due to local compression due to tamponade
- Beck's triad (minority of cases of acute cardiac tamponade):
  - Elevated JVP: Prominent x-descent, absent y-descent, Kussmaul sign (inspiratory rise in JVP)
  - Hypotension
  - Muffled heart sounds: Large pericardial effusion

- Other signs:
  - Tachycardia
  - Pulsus paradoxus (drop of systolic blood pressure by more than 10 mmHg during inspiration)—high positive predictive value and sensitivity, lower specificity
  - Pericardial rub-in cardiac tamponade due to inflammatory pericarditis

Investigations

- **ECG**
  - Sinus tachycardia, low voltage complexes (<5 mm in limb leads, <10 mm in precordial leads)
  - Look for electrical alternans: Correlates with the degree of tamponade

Chest X-ray

  - Enlarged cardiac silhouette (>200 mL of fluid). Money bag appearance with no distinct chamber enlargement
  - Pulmonary oligemia
  - To rule out mediastinal abnormalities (such as tumors)—for etiology
- Echocardiogram: Gold standard for detecting and quantifying effusion and for confirming tamponade
  - Features diagnostic of cardiac tamponade include:
    - Collapse of right atrium for > 1/3 of systole
    - Right ventricular diastolic collapse (sensitivity 48–100%; specificity 72–100%)
    - Inferior vena cava dilatation with <50% inspiratory collapse (sensitivity 97%; specificity 40%)
    - "Swinging heart": Heart moves freely in pericardial cavity with large effusion
- Additional imaging (not typically used for diagnosis, but may confirm diagnosis):
  - Cardiac CT/MRI
- Others:
  - Pericardial fluid analysis: Hematocrit level, cell count, smears, glucose level, culture, and cytology.

Differential Diagnosis

- Tension pneumothorax
- Pulmonary embolism
- Restrictive cardiomyopathy
- Constrictive pericarditis
- Right ventricular infarction

Treatment

- **Definitive therapy:** Drainage of pericardial effusion
- **Percutaneous catheter pericardiocentesis**
  - Emergency pericardiocentesis is recommended in:
    - Patients with hemodynamic instability and/or
    - Has signs of cardiac tamponade guided by echocardiography

- Preferably under echocardiography (or fluoroscopy) guidance
  - Subxiphoid approach:
    - Needle is introduced between xiphoid process and left costal margin at angle of 30–45° and directed towards left shoulder
  - Parasternal approach:
    - Needle is introduced in the left 5th intercostal space, 1 cm lateral to the sternum (to avoid internal thoracic vessels), and directed from superior to inferior rib (to avoid intercostal nerve and vessels)
    - Higher risk of pneumothorax than subxiphoid approach
  - Apical approach:
    - Not recommended in emergency.
    - Needle is introduced 1 cm lateral to the apex beat with needle angled towards right shoulder
    - Higher risk of left ventricular puncture and may precipitate ventricular fibrillation.
- Preferred for large, free-flowing effusions
- More than 1 L of effusion should not be drained, because large volume removal can precipitate left ventricular systolic failure
- Continued drainage of pericardial fluid through an indwelling catheter can prevent recurrence of neoplastic or idiopathic effusions
- Avoid if patient has:
  - Severe pulmonary hypertension
  - Uncorrected coagulopathy or currently using anticoagulant therapy use or Thrombocytopenia $< 50{,}000/mm^3$

- **Pericardiotomy—open surgical drainage**
  - Drained through a subxiphoid or apical incision
  - It is also the preferred approach in:
    - Purulent pericarditis
    - Recurrent effusions
    - When pericardial tissue is required for diagnosis
    - When the pericardial sac is not reachable with a needle
- **Percutaneous balloon pericardiotomy**
  - Percutaneous creation of a pericardial window to allow drainage of effusion into the pleural space
  - This prevents recurrence of tamponade
  - Indicated for: Tamponade caused by malignant pericardial effusions and recurrent tamponade
- Other:
  - Bedrest with legs elevated to improve venous return
  - Oxygen

- Fluid resuscitation:
  - Temporary measure for patients who are hypotensive with hypovolemic cardiac tamponade
  - However, massive fluid resuscitation may worsen tamponade
- Anti-inflammatory therapy:
  - Patients with mild tamponade may be treated with NSAIDs and/or prednisone combined with colchicine for a brief amount of time.
  - This requires vigilant, intense monitoring.
- Treatment of the underlying cause of pericardial effusion

- Therapies to avoid:
  - Inotropic agents and vasodilators
  - IV diuretics are strongly contraindicated
  - Positive pressure mechanical ventilation: May cause a sudden drop in blood pressure.

Chapter 11

Hypertensive Emergency

Definition

Elevated blood pressure (systolic pressure ≥180 and/or diastolic pressure ≥110 mmHg) having signs or symptoms of acute, ongoing target organ damage.

Evaluation

The initial evaluation is required to determine the at-risk organ and will help in guiding the management.

Signs and Symptoms

- Focal neurological deficits: Hemorrhagic/ischemic stroke
- Generalised neurologic symptoms like agitation, delirium, seizures, visual disturbances—hypertensive encephalopathy
- Chest discomfort/pain—myocardial ischemia
- Chest pain, severe backache—aortic dissection
- Oliguria—acute kidney injury
- Fundoscopy: Flame-shaped hemorrhages, cotton wool spots, papilledema—Hypertensive retinopathy

Investigations

- CT/MRI of the brain
- ECG for MI or ischemia/echo for cardiac function
- Cardiac biomarkers
- Chest X-ray for pulmonary edema
- Renal function tests
- CECT of chest or TEE—if aortic dissection is suspected

Treatment

Treat the patient, not the number. Target BP and speed of normalising BP depends on the clinical condition.

Rapid Reduction of BP Needed

1. **Acute aortic dissection:** The systolic blood pressure should be rapidly lowered to a target of 100–120 mmHg (within 20 mins)

2. **Acute pulmonary edema:** BP should be reduced as soon as possible, and with the addition of injection frusemide 40 mg IV stat and as needed. Refer to chapter on acute pulmonary edema.
3. **Eclampsia:** There is a need for urgent BP reduction here.
4. **Spontaneous intracerebral hemorrhage:**
   - Acute ICH with systolic blood pressure between 150 and 220 mmHg, lowering the BP to 140 is recommended.
   - BP >220 mmHg: Aggressive reduction of BP with continuous IV infusion to target BP between 140 and 160 mmHg.

Rapid Reduction not Advisable

Acute Ischemic Stroke

- Do not treat unless BP >220/120 mm Hg, as this will increase the size of the brain infarct, by affecting the penumbra region.
- In those who are candidates for reperfusion therapy, treat BP if it is >185/110 mmHg.

DRUG THERAPY

Nitroglycerin:

Initially 5 μg/min then titrate by 5 μg/min at 3–5 min intervals. If no response is seen at 20 μg/min then incremental doses of 10–20 μg/min may be used.

Dilution: 25 mg NTG in 45 mL NS-start at 0.6 mL/hr—titrate at doses of 0.6 mL/hr
Tolerance may develop after > 24 hr of infusion—so stop

Nitroprusside: 0.3 μg/kg/min with maximum up to 10 μg/kg/min.
Wrap the infusion bottle and drip set with aluminium foil to protect from light.

Enalaprilat: 0.625–1.25 mg over 5 min every 6–8 hours. Maximum 5 mg/dose.

Hydralazine: 10–50 mg at 30 min interval.

Labetalol: Initial bolus of 20 mg IV push over 2 mins followed by 20 to 80 mg IV bolus every 10 minutes (maximum 300 mg) until desired BP is reached or start continuous infusion 2 mg/min.

Avoid usage in asthma, COPD, HF, bradycardia or greater than first degree heart block.

Should not be used without alpha blockade in cases of pheochromocytoma, or cocaine or methamphetamine overdose.

Esmolol: 250 to 500 μg/kg loading dose over one minute; then initiate IV infusion at 25 to 50 μg/kg per minute; titrate incrementally up to maximum of 300 μg/kg per minute.

Metoprolol: 2.5–5 mg IV stat, can be repeated every 5–10 minutes, to a maximum of 15 mg.

Frusemide: Especially in patients with pulmonary edema renal failure, hypertensive encephalopathy. 40–60 mg IV STAT. Titrate to response.

Preferred Parenteral Drugs for Selected Hypertensive Emergencies

Clinical presentation	Timeline and target for BP reduction	First-line treatment	Alternative
Malignant hypertension with or without acute renal failure	Several hours reduce MAP by 20–25%	Labetalol, nicardipine	Nitroprusside
Hypertensive encephalopathy	Immediately reduce MAP by 20–25%	Labetalol, nicardipine	Nitroprusside
Acute coronary event	Immediately reduce SBP to <140 mmHg nitroglycerine, labetalol	Nitroglycerine	Labetalol
Acute cardiogenic pulmonary edema	Immediately reduce SBP to <140 mmHg	Nitroprusside or nitroglycerine (with loop diuretic)	Loop diuretic
Acute aortic dissection	Immediately reduce SBP to <120 mmHg and heart rate to <60 bpm	Esmolol and nitroprusside or nitroglycerine or nicardipine	Labetalol or metoprolol
Eclampsia and severe pre-eclampsia/HELLP	Immediately reduce SBP to <160 mmHg and DBP to <105 mmHg	Labetalol or nicardipine and magnesium sulfate	Consider delivery

Follow up:

Oral drugs must be started simultaneously to overlap with IV drugs, to ensure control of BP.

Chapter

12

Acute Pulmonary Thromboembolism

Pulmonary thromboembolism (PE) an important cause of in hospital mortality. Should be suspected in any patient who is hospitalised and deteriorates in a short period of time.

Clinical Manifestations

Source of emboli

- Deep veins of leg
- Pelvic veins
- Right sided endocarditis
- Fat-from fracture/amniotic fluid embolism

Mild to moderate sized embolism

Symptoms

- Dyspnea rest or with exertion
- Pleuritic pain—due to pulmonary infarction
- Platypnea
- Calf or thigh pain and/or swelling—due to DVT
- Hemoptysis

Signs

- Tachypnea/dyspnea—new onset, especially in hospitalised patients
- Tachycardia
- Raised JVP
- Loud P_2, RV S_3
- Deep vein thrombosis in lower limbs

Specific features of massive embolism are:

- Hemodynamic collapse
- Crushing chest pain
- Severe dyspnea/severe hypoxia

Investigations in suspected PE

Hypoxia (if massive PE)
- Low saturation by pulse oximeter
- ABG—pO_2—low, pCO_2—normal or low: Type 1 respiratory failure

CXR

- May be Normal
- May have wedge-shaped segmental opacities—pulmonary infarction
- Pleural effusion
- Oligemia of lung field in area of PE

ECG

- May be normal if PE is not massive/sub-massive
- Commonest finding is sinus tachycardia
- Right axis deviation
- RVH/RBBB
- S1, Q3, T3—specific pattern, but rare finding (6%)
- For atrial fibrillation, predisposing to PE

Biochemistry

D dimer

- Very sensitive, non-specific.
- Negative D dimer rules out PE
- Positive in sepsis, myocarditis, recent surgery, pregnancy, etc.

Routine biochemistry

- RFT
- Troponin and BNP elevated severe PE—suggest RV dysfunction

ECHO

- RV dysfunction/hypokinesia/LV D sign
- High PA pressures/TR
- Visualised clot
- Loss of inspiratory collapse in IVC

Note: A normal ECHO rules out a significant PE
Specific: **CTPA-gold standard**

- CT pulmonary angiography defines the arteries involved. Shows abrupt cut-off at site of embolism.
- 100% sensitive, 91% specific
- If CT is contraindicated, then V/Q scan can be done. Example—in renal failure/ pregnancy.

Venous Doppler

- To look for deep vein thrombosis in legs.
- Note: Several emboli come from pelvic veins, and may not be picked up by Doppler of lower limbs.

Work up for proven PE

For procoagulant state: To be sent before starting anticoagulation

- APLA screening
- Protein C, S and antithrombin III levels, homocysteinemia
- Rule out underlying connective tissue disorders/malignancy

Diagnosis and Classification

Based on 4 crucial parameters, PE is classified into high, intermediate and low risk

Risk	Hemodynamic instability	Clinical severity comorbidities	RV dysfunction	Cardiac biomarkers
High	++	++	++	++
Intermediate	–	+	+	+
Low	–	–	–	–

The probability of PE is determined based on the Wells criteria:

Clinical symptoms of DVT (pedal edema, pain on palpation)	3
Other diagnosis less likely than PE	3
Heart rate >100	1.5
Immobilization for >2 days or surgery in the previous four weeks	1.5
Previous DVT/PE	1.5
Hemoptysis	1
Malignancy	1
>6: High probability, 2–6: Moderate probability, <2: Low probability Modified Wells: >4 PE—likely, ≤4 PE—unlikely	

Management

Massive PE: BP <90 mm of Hg, hypoxia

A. Respiratory support:

1. Oxygen supplementation to maintain saturation >90%
2. Prompt consideration on intubation and mechanical ventilation in cases of respiratory failure, severe hypoxemia and hemodynamic collapse.

B. Hemodynamic support:

1. Intravenous fluid—small volumes of IV fluids usually 500–1000 mL should be given followed by vasopressor support.
2. Vasopressors: Norepinephrine is the preferred vasopressor of choice.

C. Anticoagulation: It is needed in all patients with PE. If suspicion is high, give first dose before CTPA.

Risk Factors for Bleeding

1. Age >65 years
2. Previous history of bleeding
3. Thrombocytopenia/antiplatelet therapy
4. Alcohol abuse/liver failure
5. Recent surgery

Choice of Anticoagulation

Low molecular weight heparin is preferred over UFH

Low molecular weight heparin:

- Enoxaparin: 1 mg/kg twice daily
- Dalteparin: 200 U/kg once daily
- Fondaparinux:
  - 5 mg once daily (<50 kg),
  - 7.5 mg once daily (50–100 kg),
  - 10 mg (>100 kg).

Reduced to 1.5 mg once daily in patients with creatinine clearance (CrCl) in the range of 20 to 50 mL/minute.

Unfractionated Heparin (UFH)

UFH is given as bolus and continuous IV infusion to achieve aPTT 2–3 times the upper limit of normal.

Initial dose: 80 units/kg bolus, then 18 units/kg per hour. Or 5000 units 8th hourly SC.

Definitive Therapy

Thrombolytic therapy indications

- High risk with hemodynamic instability/severe RV dysfunction/severe hypoxia/ high clot burden
- Intermediate risk with adverse clinical features
- Not responding to anticoagulation

Absolute Contraindications

1. Prior intracranial hemorrhage/intracranial neoplasm
2. Ischemic stroke within 3 months
3. Active bleeding or bleeding diathesis (excluding menses)
4. Significant head/face trauma within 3 months

Relative Contraindications

1. Severe uncontrolled hypertension (systolic >180, diastolic >110)
2. Pregnancy
3. Active peptic ulcer
4. Age >75 years
5. Current use of anticoagulant with INR >1.7 or PT(prothrombin time) >15 seconds
6. Major surgery less than 3 weeks

Thrombolytic Regimens

- Streptokinase:
  - 250,000 units over 30–60 mins followed by 100,000 units/hour for 24 hours
  - Can cause anaphylaxis.
  - Hence steroids and chlorpheniramine can be given 30 minutes before injection. Bleeding risk is also high.

- Tenecteplase: Single IV bolus
  - 60 kg—30 mg (6000 IU)
  - 60–70 kg—35 mg (7000 IU)
  - 70-80 kg—40 mg (8000 IU)
  - 80–90 kg—45 mg (9000 IU)
  - >90 kg—50 mg (10,000 IU)
- >75 years of age—reduce to half dose
- Reteplase
  - 10 units IV bolus (over 2 minutes), then
  - Second dose given 30 minutes after first (for total cumulative dose of 20 units)
  - In a dedicated line
- tPA (alteplase)—100 mg IV over 2 hours
  - In PE-related arrest, 50 mg IV bolus of tPA (alteplase) over 2 minutes.
  - Repeated after 15 minutes in the absence of return of spontaneous circulation (ROSC).
- Urokinase: 4400 units/kg IV over 10mins followed by 4400 units/kg/hour for 12 hours.

Interventions

- Catheter directed thrombolysis can be tried in patients not responding to above measures.
- Embolectomy: In patients who have contraindications for thrombolysis, or do not respond to catheter directed thrombolysis also.

For patients with sub-massive and mild PE

LMWH, followed by oral anticoagulants will suffice.

Choice of Anticoagulation

- All patients with PE will require anticoagulation for prevention of recurrence.
- This should be started after parenteral anticoagulation for the first 5–10 days.

Novel Oral Anticoagulants (NOACs)

These are preferred over warfarin. Have proven better efficacy, and do not need PT monitoring.

Direct thrombin inhibitors: Dabigatran 150 mg twice daily

Xa inhibitors

- Apixaban 10 mg bd (for first seven days) followed by 5 mg bd.
- Rivaroxaban 15 mg bd for first three weeks followed by 20 mg od, for 6 months, followed by 10 mg od later.

Note

Rivaroxaban and apixaban can be started without parenteral anticoagulation.Dabigatran needs to be given only after parenteral anticoagulation is done.

Vit K Antagonists

It is preferred over NOACs in the following conditions: Pregnancy/renal failure/ APLA syndrome

Warfarin

- 5–10 mg daily to target a PT/INR of 2–2.5.
- In APLA, target can be raised to 2.5–3.5

Acenocoumarol

- 1–10 mg adjust to target PT INR

Anticoagulation in Pregnancy with PE

- 0–12 weeks—LMWH
- 12 to 36 weeks warfarin
- After 36 weeks—LMWH
- UFH during delivery

Dose Adjustment in Renal Failure

Drug	GFRml/min	Dose
Dabigatran	<50	110 mg bd, do not use below <30 mL
Rivaroxaban	<50 mL	15 mg od
Apixaban	Age > 80, cr >1.5 mg/dL, wt <60 kg (any 2 of these)	2.5 mg bd

No dose adjustment needed for warfarin/acenocoumarol in renal failure

Duration of Therapy

- For patients with PE—minimum of 6 months full dose.
- Can deescalate to lower doses after 6 months and given up to 12 months.
- For patients with procoagulant state and malignancy—lifelong

IVC filters

- Patients with absolute contraindication to anticoagulant therapy (e.g. hemorrhagic stroke, significant active bleeding
- Patients with massive PE who survived but in whom recurrent embolism is possible and may be fatal
- Patients who develop recurrent venous thromboembolism in spite of adequate anticoagulant treatment.
- Retrievable or permanent filters can be placed according to patient's clinical indication.

Chapter

13

Myocarditis

- It is an inflammatory disease of cardiac muscle.
- It can be acute, subacute or chronic

Causes of Myocarditis

Infectious causes	Non-infectious causes
• Viral (most common) ◆ Dengue ◆ Influenza A and B ◆ Coxsackie B ◆ Covid 19 • Bacterial ◆ Tuberculosis ◆ Staphylococcal, pneumococcal ◆ Scrub typhus, mycoplasma • Spirochetal—leptospirosis • Protozoal ◆ Malaria	• Cardiotoxins ◆ Alcohol ◆ Cocaine • Systemic diseases ◆ Collagen vascular disease • Hypersensitivity reaction ◆ Snake bite ◆ Insect bites (wasp, bee, spider, scorpion) • Radiation

Clinical Manifestations

Acute myocarditis presents in 1–2 weeks after the inciting event .
The clinical profile

- ACS like syndrome–
- New onset or worsening heart failure, cardiogenic shock
- Arrhythmias

Symptoms

- Chest pain—retrosternal
- Sudden onset breathlessness
- Palpitations
- Fatigue, dizziness

Signs

- Unexplained tachycardia/bradycardia/irregular pulse/tachypnea
- Elevated JVP/bilateral basal crepitations/S_3 S_4 gallop

Investigations

- Cardiac biomarkers—serial elevation of troponin T
- NTproBNP may be elevated in patients presenting as heart failure or cardiogenic shock
- ECG—may show: Non-specific changes
  - Sinus tachycardia
  - Diffuse T wave inversion/nonspecific ST segment changes—not wall specific
  - QRS/QT prolongation/ventricular arrhythmias
  - AV conduction blocks
- Echocardiogram—regional or global left ventricular dysfunction
- Chest X-ray—acute pulmonary edema
- Coronary angiogram—if done, will show normal vessels

Management

It is usually nonspecific and is guided based on the clinical presentation of myocarditis.

- Treat CCF/Cardiogenic shock/arrhythmias (refer to chapters on these topics).
- Treatment of the underlying cause is the most effective.

Other supportive measures:

- Bedrest—initially
- Salt and fluid restriction
- Maintain heart rate less than 100/min—consider ivabradine 5–7.5 mg bd (for patients with sinus tachycardia) or beta-blockers for the same
- Diuretics and inotropes—refer to Chapter 3: Management Acute Decompensated Heart Failure and Pulmonary Edema.

Therapies which have been tried (efficacy uncertain)

- Viral myocarditis: Ribavirin or interferon alpha
- Immunosuppressive therapy—in collagen vascular disease, sarcoidosis, giant cell myocarditis, eosinophilic myocarditis
- Dosage: Methylprednisolone—1 mg/kg for 4 weeks and then tapered. Azathioprine—100 to 150 mg daily can be added.
- IV immunoglobulins (IVIg) in myocarditis—doubtful use

Patients presenting with myocarditis usually have a prolonged hospital/ICU stay with a poorer prognosis.

Chapter

14

Aortic Dissection

Classification

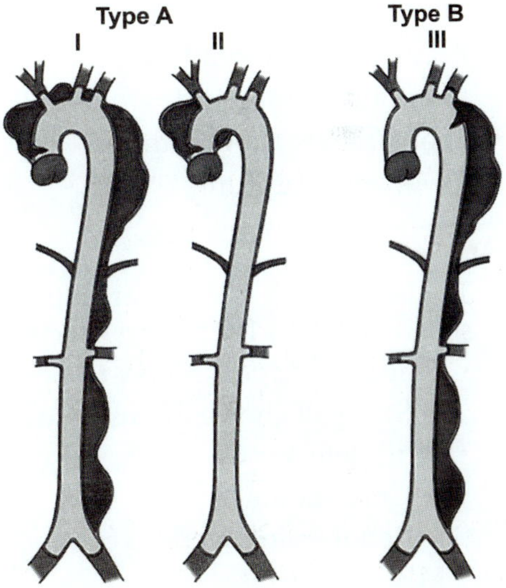

- Stanford (more commonly used):
  - Type A: Ascending aorta
  - Type B: Descending aorta
- DeBakey:
  - Type I: Ascending and descending aorta
  - Type II: Ascending aorta
  - Type III: Descending aorta
- Based on duration of presentation:
  - Hyperacute: <24 hr
  - Acute: 2 to 7 days
  - Subacute: 8 to 30 days
  - Chronic: >30 days

Risk Factors

- Hypertension
- Genetic: Marfan syndrome, Ehlers-Danlos syndrome, Turner syndrome.
- Bicuspid aortic valve (including prior aortic valve replacement)/coarctation of aorta.
- Vasculitis: Takayasu arteritis, giant cell arteritis, Behçet's syndrome, ankylosing spondylitis.

Clinical Features

- *Pain:* Sudden onset of severe sharp, ripping, tearing, or stabbing pain located in chest (ascending aorta-common), back (descending), neck(arch) and/or abdomen (less common)
- Syncope/hemiparesis
- *Dyspnea*—with features of left ventricular failure
- Asymmetric, decreased, or absent peripheral pulses
- *Blood pressure:*
  - Differential blood pressure >20 mmHg between arms
  - Hypertension may be present

- 25% present with hypotension—indicates bleeding, cardiac tamponade, or severe aortic regurgitation, indicating bad prognosis.
- *Auscultation:*
  - Diastolic decrescendo murmur—aortic regurgitation
  - New-onset pericardial friction rubs—pericarditis or pericardial effusion
- *Reduced organ perfusion:*
  - Myocardial ischemia
  - Stroke
  - Mesenteric ischemia
  - Acute kidney injury

Differential Diagnosis

- Acute coronary syndrome
- Pulmonary embolism
- Spontaneous pneumothorax
- Esophageal rupture

Investigations

- Transesophageal echocardiography, multidetector CT, and MRI are all highly sensitive (98 to 100%) and specific (95 to 98%).
  - Transesophageal echocardiography (TEE)
    - Study of choice in unstable patients with type A dissection
  - Multidetector CT
    - Gold standard
    - Requires intravenous contrast—use may be limited in patients with renal failure
  - MRI
    - Not suitable for unstable patients
- Others:
  - Chest X-ray
    - Widened superior mediastinum with abnormal aortic contour
  - ECG:
    - To rule out STEMI.
    - May show LVH, myocardial ischemia
  - Soluble ST_2 concentration: Elevated soluble ST_2 concentration—high sensitivity and moderate specificity for diagnosing acute aortic dissection

Management

- Proximal dissections (acute Stanford type A) require emergent surgery to prevent rupture or pericardial effusion.
- Distal dissections (Stanford type B) are usually treated medically unless distal organ involvement or impending rupture occurs.
  - Thoracic endovascular aortic repair (TEVAR) recommended if any complications:
    - Persistent or recurrent pain

- Refractory hypertension
- Early aortic expansion
- Malperfusion syndromes (such as visceral, renal, or limb perfusion), or
- Signs of rupture

- Open surgical repair recommended for patients with chronic dissection and aneurysm >5.5 cm but without comorbid disease

- Medical management of acute aortic dissection:
  - Intubate and ventilate without delay if profound hemodynamic instability
  - Maintain mean arterial blood pressure ≥70 mm Hg and euvolemia
    - IV fluid boluses/If unresponsive after fluid bolus, give IV vasopressor
  - Medications for stable patients (no hypotension or cardiogenic shock)
  - Rate-control:
    - Target heart rate ≤60 beats/minute
    - IV beta-blockers, if no contraindications.
      - Labetalol:
        - Bolus doses of 20–80 mg at 10-minute intervals until target blood pressure reached
        - Infusion of 0.5–2 mg/minute, adjusted until target BP is achieved
      - Esmolol:
        - Loading dose 0.5 mg/kg over 2–5 minutes
        - Followed by 0.1–0.2 mg/kg/minute infusion (maximum 0.3 mg/kg/minute)
      - Propranolol: 0.05–0.15 mg/kg every 4–6 hours
    - If contraindication to beta-blockers—use verapamil
  - Vasodilators:
    - After adequate heart rate control
    - IV enalaprilat/sodium nitroglycerine/nicardipine to reduce BP
  - Pain relief: Morphine IV 2–10 mg IV, if BP >100 mm of Hg
- Chronic management
  - Aggressive blood pressure control: Target <120/80 mm Hg
  - Statin therapy to reduce low-density lipoprotein <70 mg/dL
  - Lifestyle modifications: Tobacco cessation, minimize strenuous physical activity such as heavy lifting.
  - Serial imaging of the aorta, with multidetector CT or MRI should be performed at presentation, at 1, 3, 6, and 12 months.Endovascular repair should be considered when
    - Aortic diameter exceeds 5.5 cm
    - Uncontrolled pain or uncontrolled blood pressure, or
    - There is rapid growth of the dissecting aneurysm (>4 mm per yr)

Section

2

Neurology

Chapter

15

Cerebrovascular Accident

Abrupt onset of a focal neurological deficit that is attributable to a vascular cause.

Cerebrovascular accident (CVA) can be of the following types:

a. Ischemic (85%)
   - Thrombotic
   - Embolic

b. Hemorrhagic stroke (15%)

Anterior circulation stroke

Look for FAST symptoms

- Face: Any facial asymmetry
- Arm: Any limb weakness
- Speech: Look for dysarthria
- Time: Onset of deficits to be noticed for option of thrombolysis

Posterior circulation stroke

Dysarthria, **d**ysphagia, **d**izziness, **d**iplopia, **d**eterioration of consciousness and **a**taxia.

Vital signs: Look for

- Pulse
  - Atrial fibrillation (embolic stroke)
  - Bradycardia—raised intracranial tension
- BP: If high, could be essential hypertension or reactive
- Respiratory rate: Watch for tachypnea, Cheyne-Stokes or Biot's breathing, check O_2 saturation
- Temperature: For fever.

CNS

- Grade consciousness by Glasgow Coma Scale. Low GCS indicates large infarct in cortex, or brainstem involvement
- Pupils: Anisocoria may indicate raised ICT and coning
- 6th nerve palsy in case of raised ICT
- UMN 7th nerve palsy: Internal capsule lesions
- Focal neurological deficit: Hemiplegia monoplegia
- Cerebellar signs: Posterior circulation strokes.

Important differential diagnosis

- Transient ischemic attack (TIA) (related but is managed differently)
- Postictal paralysis
- Hypoglycemia: Neuroglycopenia
- Brain tumor or abscess
- Cerebral venous thrombosis
- PRES (posterior reversible encephalopathy syndrome)

DIAGNOSIS OF STROKE

Investigations

- Routine: Blood sugar, renal function tests, Na^+, K^+, CBP, PT/INR.
- ABG if patient is breathless
- ECG: For LVH, IHD/AF
- ECHO: For wall motion abnormalities, EF, and clots
- Holter monitoring: To screen for atrial fibrillation and other cardiac arrhythmias

Imaging of Brain

a. Computed tomography—**gold standard** for diagnosis of an **intracranial hemorrhage**.
b. *Note:* In ischemic stroke, CT done in the first 6 hours may be normal.
   - Earliest CT changes in an ischemic stroke are loss of gray matter and white matter differentiation.
   - Insular Ribbon sign—hypodensity and swelling of the insular cortex. It is a subtle early CT—sign of infarction in the territory of the middle cerebral artery.
   - After 48 hours a well demarcated wedge shaped opacity in the affected vascular territory seen.
   - Watch for **middle cerebral artery dense sign (blue arrow)** which signifies the presence of thrombus, seen in 2–6 hours **(Fig. 15.1)**.

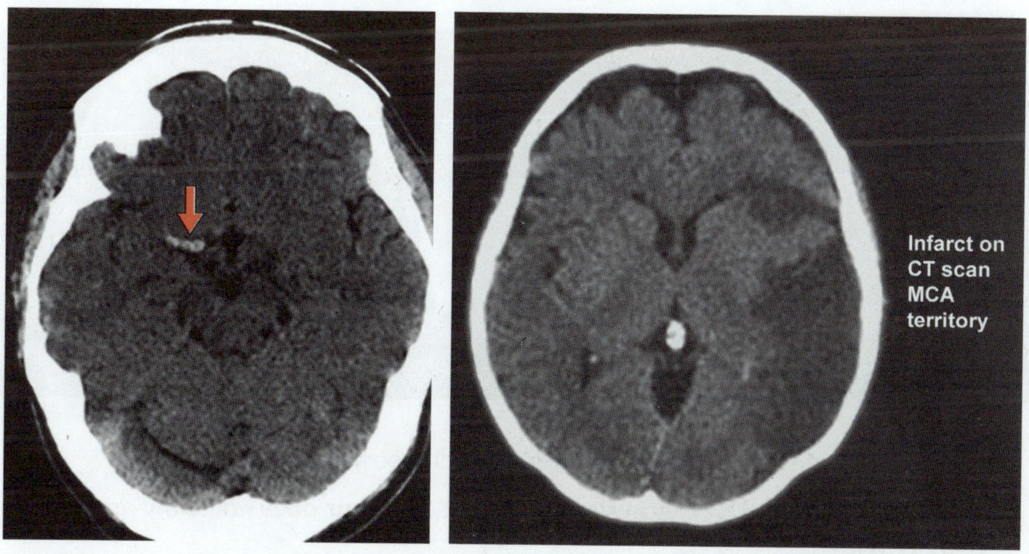

Fig. 15.1: Large infarct in MCA territory. Blue arrow shows MCA dense sign

- MCA dot sign signifies the presence of thrombus in MCA.
- ASPECTS score: The Alberta stroke program early CT score (ASPECTS) is a 10-point quantitative topographic CT scan score used in patients with middle cerebral artery stroke.
- CT perfusion studies available at a few centers help to demarcate the ischemic penumbra which is potentially salvageable if immediate measures like thrombolysis are undertaken **(Fig. 15.2A to C)**.

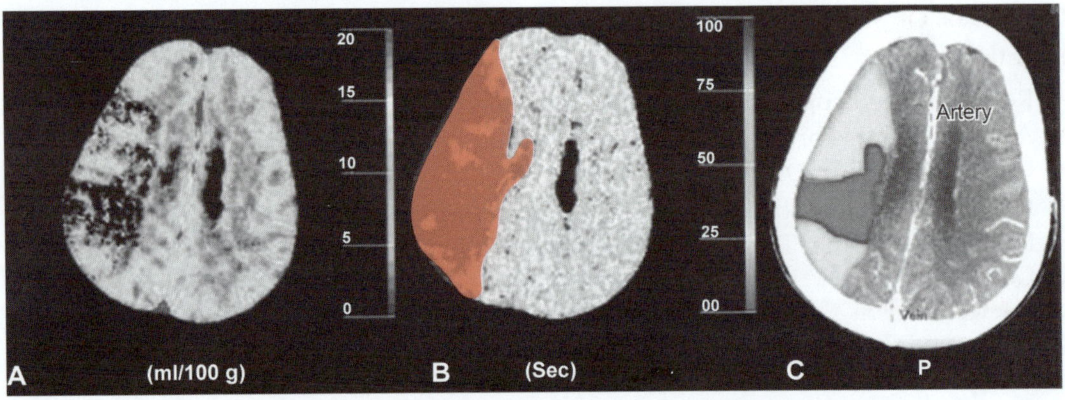

Fig. 15.2A to C: Ischemic penumbra (black in A, blue in B, white in C)

c. MRI studies

- A MRI stroke protocol study comprises 3 images primarily T2 Flair, diffusion weighted imaging and apparent diffusion coefficient.
- These help to delineate the infarcted tissue from the potentially salvageable ischemic penumbra.
- An acute infarct is seen as a bright spot in DWI and a dark spot in ADC **(Fig. 15.3)**.

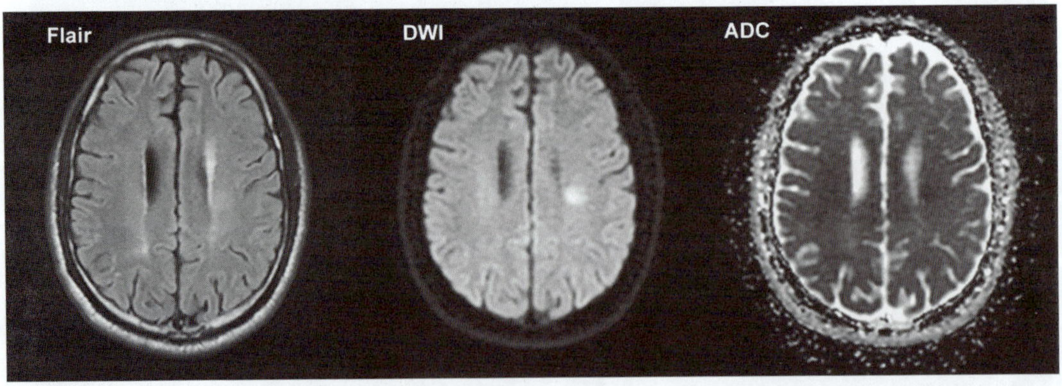

Fig. 15.3: DWI showing bright spot in early infarction

- In early infarction, DWI shows a bright spot and Flair does not show any change **(Fig. 15.4)**.

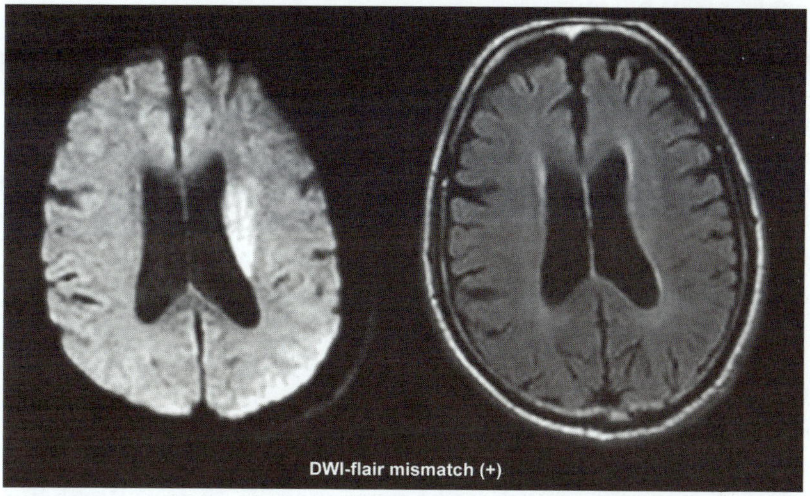

Fig. 15.4: Image on right is DW showing infarct. Image on right is flair showing no change

d. Carotid vertebral Doppler: The patency, flow velocities in the carotid and vertebral arteries should be assessed for intervention purposes.
e. CT or MR angiography should be done to identify the affected artery.

TREATMENT OF ACUTE ISCHEMIC STROKE

a. Medical support
b. Thrombolysis
c. Endovascular revascularization
d. Antithrombotic treatment/anticoagulation
e. Neuroprotection
f. Stroke rehabilitation

MEDICAL MANAGEMENT

Management of unconscious patient (for more details, refer to Chapter 23: Coma)

- Endotracheal intubation in case the patient cannot keep airway patent/saturation <90% on room air/if GCS <7.
- Control sugars, and maintain sugar levels between 110 mg/dL and 180 mg/dL. Avoid hypoglycemia.
- Treat fever aggressively, as it increases metabolic demand of brain.
- IV fluids: Avoid hypotonic solutions such as 5D or DNS, as they increase cerebral edema
- Insert Ryle's tube and Foley's catheter.
- Deep venous thrombosis prophylaxis—heparin 5000 IU SC bd, Mechanical DVT prophylaxis
- Ulcer prophylaxis with PPIs
- Watch for infections like aspiration pneumonia, urinary tract infection and skin infections.
- Treat seizure as recommended

BLOOD PRESSURE MANAGEMENT

BP should be brought down gradually in an ischemic stroke, as fast reduction in BP will decrease cerebral blood flow and increase penumbra of stroke.

- Blood pressure to be treated only if >220/120 mm Hg.
- If BP needs to be lowered for other reasons (e.g. pulmonary edema), 15% reduction every 24 hours can be done. Gradual reduction over one week to target of 140/90 mm Hg.
- In case of thrombolysis needed should be decreased to <185/110 mm Hg.
- Preferred drugs: Amlodipine and beta blockers.

TREATMENT OF ICT

- Raised ICT peaks at 48–72 hours after stroke.
- Look for CT/MRI evidence of edema.
- Raise head end at 30 degrees.
- For ICT, start IV mannitol 100 mL (to be given over 10–15 min) IV 8th hourly; target serum osmolality: 320 mOsmol/L. Avoid in renal failure/pulmonary edema.
- 3% saline boluses of 100–200 mL can be given with target Na of 155 mEq/dL.
- IV frusemide 20 mg IV 8th hourly (weak effect).
- Oral glycerol 15–30 mL tid through RT.
- Intubation and hyperventilation with target CO_2 of 25–30 mm Hg, for 24–36 hours
- Therapeutic hypothermia (around 32°C).
- Vasopressor therapy to increase mean arterial pressure if needed to improve cerebral perfusion pressure in ICT.

  Neurosurgery opinion to be sought for hemicraniectomy and other decompression surgeries if required.

Indications for Neurosurgical Intervention

- Within 48 hours of stroke onset
- Patients age ≤60 years
- Malignant hemispheric infarction (>50 percent infarction of MCA territory by CT/MRI +ACA/PCA infarction)
- Signs of impending coning like anisocoria/bradycardia
- For better survival chances—neurological deficit may persist. Patients' relatives have to be told about pros and cons.

THROMBOLYSIS

- Alteplase 0.9 mg/kg (maximum dose of 90 mg), 10% bolus and remainder as an infusion in 100 ml normal saline over 1 hour.
- Timing: Up to **3–4.5 hours after** the onset of stroke (NINDS trial/ECAS III trial). In wake up strokes, to go by MRI picture of DW positive and flair negative (<6 hours).
- Indications for thrombolysis
  1. Clinical impression of stroke
  2. Age >18 years
  3. Onset of stroke less than 4.5 hours ago
  4. No edema or hemorrhage of more than 1/3rd of the MCA territory

Contraindications for thrombolysis in stroke

- Recent MI
- BP >185/110 mm Hg
- Platelets <100,000/increased INR
- Surgery in the last 2 weeks/GI bleed in last 3 weeks/stroke or head injury in last 3 months
- Rapidly improving stroke
- NIHSS score >22 (refer to Table 15.1), avoid thrombolysis due to increased chances of hemorrhagic transformation

- **Immediate endovascular revascularization-thrombectomy**
  - Occlusion of larger vessels like MCA, ICA fails to open with thrombolysis due to large clot volume.
  - PROACT2 trial showed use of intra-arterial administration of pro-urokinase
  - Mechanical thrombectomy: Up to 8 hours after onset (MERCI trial)/DAWN and DEFUSE-3 trial: up to 16–24 hours

  Long-term intervention for prevention
  - Carotid atherosclerosis
    - Symptomatic carotid stenosis of >50% (or)
    - Asymptomatic stenosis > 70% on digital subtraction angiography may undergo-
      A. Carotid endarterectomy (>70 yr of age), or
      B. Angioplasty with stenting (<70 yr)
- **Antithrombotic treatment**
  - Aspirin 150 mg for 4 weeks (CAST trial)
  - Clopidogrel (75 mg) and Aspirin (150 mg) for 3 weeks (CHANCE and POINT trial)
  - Statins: Atorvastatin 40 mg/day for 4 weeks, tapered over 6 months to 10 mg/day.

  Anticoagulation: For
  1. Atrial fibrillation
  2. Basilar artery thrombosis
  3. Impending carotid artery occlusion
  4. Mural thrombus
  5. Prior embolic phenomenon
- **Neuroprotection** (doubtful use)
  Hypothermia for 24 hours to slow the metabolism, decrease the infarct.
  Piracetam 800 mg tid
- **Rehabilitation**
  - Physiotherapy—after 24 hours
  - Speech therapy
  - Occupational therapy

TREATMENT OF EMBOLIC STROKE

Management is same as thrombotic stroke
Define source: Cardiac—by echo, carotids—by Doppler

Anticoagulation

- IV enoxaparin 1 mg/kg bd for 5 days,
- Overlap with NOACs or warfarin after day 2.
- Target INR is 2–3.
- Treatment may be lifelong for those with continuing embolic risk
- Contraindicated in large infarcts and patients with infective endocarditis

ACUTE INTRACRANIAL HEMORRHAGE

- Most important risk factor:
  - Essential hypertension
  - In young adults: Aneurysms or arteriovenous malformations
- Typical sites of hypertensive bleed: Basal ganglia, cerebellum, pons, then lobar.
- *A lobar bleed should always raise the possibility of aneurysm/AVM*
- Symptoms: Headache, vomiting, convulsions, coma
- Signs: Unconsciousness and focal deficits

Investigation

CT is the gold standard for hemorrhage.

In case of intracranial hemorrhage, intraventricular extension, volume of the bleed and presence of midline shift should be looked for.

INTRACRANIAL HEMORRHAGE SCORE

Components: Age, hematoma volume, intraventricular extension and infratentorial source of bleed (Fig. 15.5).

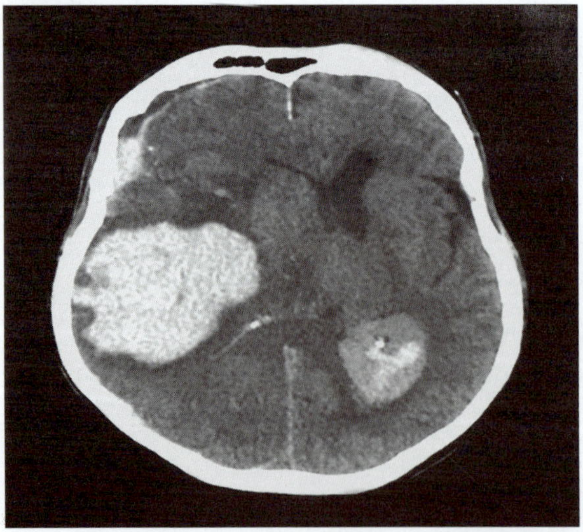

Fig. 15.5: Right cerebral bleed with intraventricular extension and midline shift

TREATMENT

- Stabilize the patient by maintaining airway and breathing
- Withhold anti-platelets and anticoagulants

- ***Maintain BP <140 mm of Hg systolic***. Cerebral perfusion pressure between 50 and 70 mm Hg (interact 2 trial)
- Anticonvulsants in patients with seizures: IV levetiracetam 1 gm bd.
- No role for prophylactic anticonvulsants. Seizures more common in lobar bleeds.
- ICH score must be calculated.
- **Neurosurgery opinion:** Indications are:
  - *Decompression surgeries:*
    - Infratentorial bleed: Cerebellar >3 cm/with neurological deterioration
    - Supratentorial accessible lobar bleed >2 cm with GCS >5
  - *Ventricular drainage*
    - For obstructive hydrocephalus due to intraventricular extension of hemorrhage.

Table 15.1: NIHSS Scale in Stroke

1a. Level of consciousness	0 = Alert; keenly responsive 1 = Not alert; but arousable by minor stimulation 2 = Not alert; requires repeated stimulation 3 = Unresponds or responds only with reflex
1b. Level of consciousness questions: What is your age? What is the month?	0 = Answers two questions correctly 1 = Answers one question correctly 2 = Answers neither questions correctly
1c. Level of consciousness commands: Open and close your eyes Grip and release your hand	0 = Performs both tasks correctly 1 = Performs one task correctly 2 = Performs neither task correctly
2. Best gaze	0 = NormalW 1 = Partial gaze palsy 2 = Forced deviation
3. Visual	0 = No visual lost 1 = Partial hemianopia 2 = Complete hemianopia 3 = Bilateral hemianopia
4. Facial palsy	0 = Normal symmetric movements 1 = Minor paralysis 2 = Partial paralysis 3 = Complete paralysis of one or both sides
5. Motor arm: Left arm Right arm	0 = No drift 1 = Drift 2 = Some effort against gravity 3 = No effort against gravity 4 = No movement
6. Motor leg: Left leg Right leg	0 = No drift 1 = Drift 2 = Some effort against gravity 3 = No effort against gravity 4 = No movement

Contd.

Table 15.1: NIHSS Scale in Stroke (Contd.)	
7. Limb ataxia	0 = Absent 1 = Present in one limb 2 = Present in two limb
8. Sensory	0 = Normal; no sensory loss 1 = Mild-to-moderate sensory loss 2 = Severe-to-total sensory loss
9. Best language	0 = No aphasia; normal 1 = Mild-to-moderate aphasia 2 = Severe aphasia 3 = Mute; global aphasia
10. Dysarthria	0 = Normal 1 = Mild-to-moderate dysarthria 2 = Severe dysarthria
11. Extinction and inattention	0 = No abnormality 1 = Visual, tactile, auditory, spatial, or personal inattention 2 = Profound hemi-inattention or extinction
Score = 0–42	

Chapter 16

Subarachnoid Hemorrhage

Causes

1. Rupture of saccular aneurysm
2. Arteriovenous malformations
3. Extension from intracerebral hemorrhage
4. Head trauma

CLINICAL FEATURES

Symptoms

1. Headache—**sudden onset**, severe headache–described as "worst headache of my life" often called **thunderclap headache**.
2. Loss of consciousness
3. Neck pain/stiffness
4. Vomiting
5. Seizures
6. "Sentinel headache"—severe sudden headache weeks prior to major Subarachnoid hemorrhage (SAH): It may represent either a minor hemorrhage (a "warning leak") or physical changes within the aneurysm wall (e.g. acute dissection, thrombosis, or expansion).

Findings	Cause
Neck stiffness	Meningeal irritation
Third nerve palsy	Posterior communicating, posterior cerebral, superior cerebellar aneurysm
Sixth nerve palsy	Elevated ICP (false localising sign)
Ophthalmoplegia	Internal carotid artery aneurysm impinging on cavernous sinus
Unilateral visual loss or bitemporal hemianopia	Internal carotid aneurysm compressing optic nerve/ optic chiasma
Brainstem signs	Basilar artery aneurysm

Contd.

Findings	Cause
Hemiparesis and aphasia or visuospatial neglect	Middle cerebral artery aneurysm, parenchymal hematomas
Bilateral leg weakness and abulia	Anterior communicating artery aneurysm
Impaired level of consciousness and impaired upward gaze	Hydrocephalus with pressure on dorsal midbrain
Retinal and subhyaloid hemorrhages	SAH leak into retina
Pre-retinal hemorrhages (Terson syndrome)	Vitreous hemorrhage due to raised ICP

Hunt and Hess Grading of SAH

Grade	Neurological Feature
Grade 1	Asymptomatic or mild headache and slight nuchal rigidity
Grade 2	Severe headache, neck stiffness, no neurological deficit except cranial nerve palsy
Grade 3	Somnolent, confused, focal neurological deficits
Grade 4	Stuporous, severe hemiparesis
Grade 5	Coma, decerebrate posturing

DIAGNOSIS

All patients with headache characterized as sudden, rapid onset of severe headache should be evaluated for SAH.

Investigations

- Non-contrast CT of the brain. Sensitivity—100% when CT is done within 6 hours of the onset of headache. Sensitivity decreases to 50% after one week.
- Look for blood in the basal cisterns, sylvian fissures, interhemispheric fissures, suprasellar cisterns. Intracerebral extension is present in 20–40% of patients **(Fig. 16.1)**.

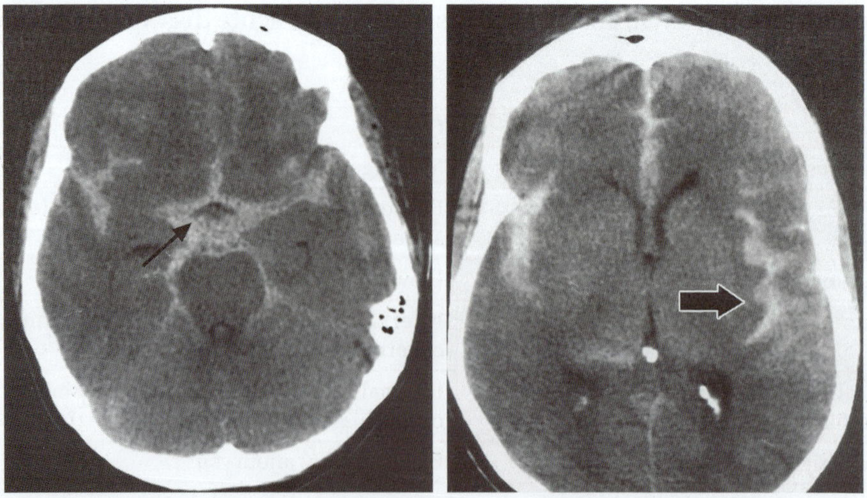

Fig. 16.1: CT scan shows blood in the subarachnoid space, suggesting SAH

LUMBAR PUNCTURE (LP)

Not needed if CT already shows SAH.

LP is mandatory if there is strong suspicion of SAH, when CT brain is normal.

May show

- Raised opening pressure
- Elevated RBC count
- Xanthochromia

How to Differentiate the Traumatic CSF from SAH in LP?

- Three tube test: No decline in RBC count in successive test tubes with CSF is suggestive of SAH.
- The greater RBC count in the last tube is more suggestive of SAH.
- Higher RBC/WBC ratio (in blood is 700 to 1000:1.)

TO IDENTIFY THE SOURCE OF BLEEDING

Digital Subtraction Angiography (DSA) is the gold standard investigation and has the best resolution for identifying an aneurysm.

Patients with negative angiography: A repeat angiography is essential 4–14 days after the initial scan and a DSA is recommended

Non-aneurysmal SAH: 15–20% of SAH have non-aneurysmal causes like

- Intracranial arterial dissection
- Vascular malformations
- Perimesencephalic hemorrhage
- CVT
- Traumatic SAH
- CNS tumors

MANAGEMENT

- Initial–stabilizing the patient and securing airway, breathing and circulation
- Definitive treatment of SAH
  - Early repair of aneurysm by surgical clipping or endovascular coiling.
  - Surgery for aneurysm

Medical Management

1. **Blood pressure maintenance:** Should be maintained around an ideal range on a case to case basis.
   - Avoid hypotension. BP is needed for cerebral perfusion (cerebral perfusion pressure). If it is low, it will cause infarction of the brain by compromising cerebral blood flow.
   - For most patients with acute SAH, the goal is to maintain SBP <160 mm Hg or MAP <110 mm Hg. Use pre-SAH blood pressure as guide.
   - Intravenous labetalol, nicardipine, or enalapril are preferred and vasodilators like nitroglycerin and nitroprusside should be avoided.

2. **Maintaining euvolemia:** To avoid cerebral ischemia and treat vasospasm
   - IV NS to avoid hypovolemia—this can cause infarction.
   - IV vasopressors—can also be used usually—norepinephrine or phenylephrine
   - Watch for SIADH (very common) or cerebral salt wasting.
   - Both cause hyponatremia—recognize and treat.
3. **Nimodipine—for vasospasm:** To be started within 48 hours—60 mg every 4 hours and continued for 21 days.
   Close BP monitoring should be done.

Other Supportive Measures

1. **Seizure prophylaxis:** Levetiracetam: Loading dose 20 mg/kg followed by maintenance of 1 gm every 12 hours (maximum 1.5 gm 12 hourly)
2. **Raised ICP**
   a. CSF diversion—external ventricular drain is indicated in patients with worsening sensorium with evidence of raised ICP/hydrocephalus
   b. Osmotic therapy and diuresis—hypertonic saline, acetazolamide
   c. Hemicraniectomy
3. **Pain control:** Acetaminophen 500 mg every 3–4 hours and for severe pain opiates like tramadol and morphine can be used.
4. **DVT prophylaxis:** Mechanical DVT prophylaxis is preferred

Management of Complications

1. Rebleeding from aneurysm:
   - Most often occurs in first 2–24 hours
   - Measures taken to prevent rebleeding include:
     - Bedrest in a quiet room
     - Analgesia and sedation.
     - Stool softeners: To prevent rise in BP and ICT
   - Treatment is early surgery to clip aneurysm
2. Cerebral infarction due to vasospasm causing infarction:
   - It usually occurs at 4–14 days after rupture of aneurysm and peak at 7 days
   - Present with deficits like hemiplegia, aphasia, loss of consciousness
   - Patient may need repeat CT at this time to document infarction
3. Acute hydrocephalus—ventricular drainage

Prognosis

Features suggesting poor prognosis: Increasing age, poor initial level of consciousness and large SAH.

Chapter

17

Cerebral Venous Thrombosis

- Thrombosis of the venous channels in the brain is an uncommon cause of cerebral infarction.
- Has potential mortality.

Risk Factors—Prothrombotic States

1. **Pregnancy/puerperium**
2. Drugs (oral contraceptives, hormone replacement therapy)
3. Hematologic conditions (hypercoagulable)
    - Paroxysmal nocturnal hemoglobinuria (PNH)
    - **Polycythemia**
    - Protein C deficiency/protein S deficiency
    - Antithrombin III deficiency/factor V Leiden mutation/G20210 prothrombin mutation
    - **APLA syndrome**
    - Hyperhomocysteinemia
    - Myeloproliferative neoplasms
4. Head injury
5. Infection (CNS infections, local infections of the paranasal sinus, ear)
6. Malignancy involving CNS
7. Idiopathic (13%)
8. Inflammatory diseases (SLE, Behcet disease, granulomatosis polyangiitis, sarcoidosis, inflammatory bowel disease)

Clinical features: They are grouped under three syndromes:

1. **Isolated intracranial hypertension syndrome**
    - **Headache:** Most common complaint, localized or diffuse, gradual or sudden in onset
    - Papilledema or visual disturbances may be present.
    - ***Any undiagnosed severe headache, with no obvious cause, cerebral venous thrombosis (CVT) should be ruled out.***
2. **Focal syndrome:** Stroke with monoparesis, paraplegia, hemiparesis or seizures
3. **Encephalopathy:** Altered levels of consciousness, cognitive dysfunction, stupor or coma

Features according to individual sinus thrombosis

Cavernous sinus thrombosis	Orbital pain, chemosis, proptosis, 3, 4, 6th nerve palsies
Sagittal sinus thrombosis	Motor deficits with bilateral involvement, seizures
Jugular vein/lateral sinus thrombosis	Pulsating tinnitus
Isolated lateral sinus thrombosis	Headache, rarely aphasia (motor type)
Lateral sinus, jugular, posterior fossa veins	Multiple cranial nerve palsies
Deep cerebral venous system—straight sinus and its branches	Severe encephalopathy like presentation

When to suspect CVT?

1. Cerebral infarction not restricted to arterial boundaries
2. Hemorrhagic stroke of unclear origin
3. **A headache where routine CT/MRI is normal**
4. Clinical risk: Pregnancy, OC pills, hypercoagulable state

URGENT IMAGING

Urgent MRI-brain with MR-venography (or if MRI not possible CT with CT venography).

Imaging	Findings
CT-brain (Fig. 17.1)	• May be normal in about 30% cases. • Hemorrhagic infarcts • Dense triangle sign (hyperdensity, triangle shape in posterior part of superior sagittal sinus) • Empty delta sign (In CECT seen as a triangle with central part lacking the contrast due to thrombus in the posterior part of superior sagittal sinus) • Cord sign (CECT—a linear hyperdensity seen over the cerebral cortex due to thrombosed vein) • Indirect signs—contrast enhancement of falx and tentorium, dilated cerebral veins and small ventricles. • Hemorrhagic infarcts
MRI-brain (Fig. 17.2)	Depends on the age of the thrombus the thrombosed sinus appears 1. <5 days—isointense on T_1 and hypointense on T_2 2. >5 days—hyperintense on both T_1 and T_2 3. >1month—variable pattern, may appear isointense Secondary brain lesions such as cerebral edema, hemorrhagic infarcts.
MR-venography (Fig. 17.3)	**Most specific:** Absence of flow in the cerebral venous sinuses

Evaluation for thrombophilic state

- An evaluation for thrombophilic state: Antiphospholipid, lupus anticoagulant, anti-cardiolipin antibodies, protein S, protein C, antithrombin III, and Leiden factor V mutation.

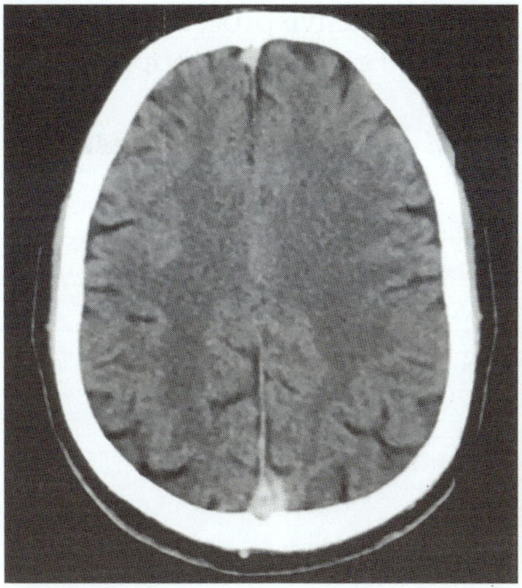

Fig. 17.1: CT-brain—Dense delta sign

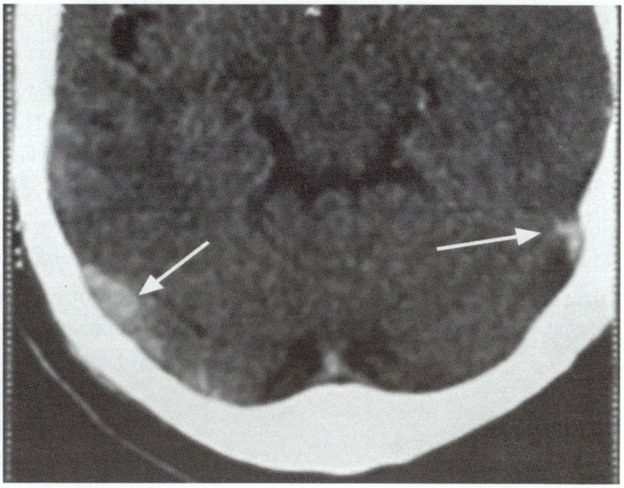

Fig. 17.2: Intense contrast enhancement of falx, tentorium

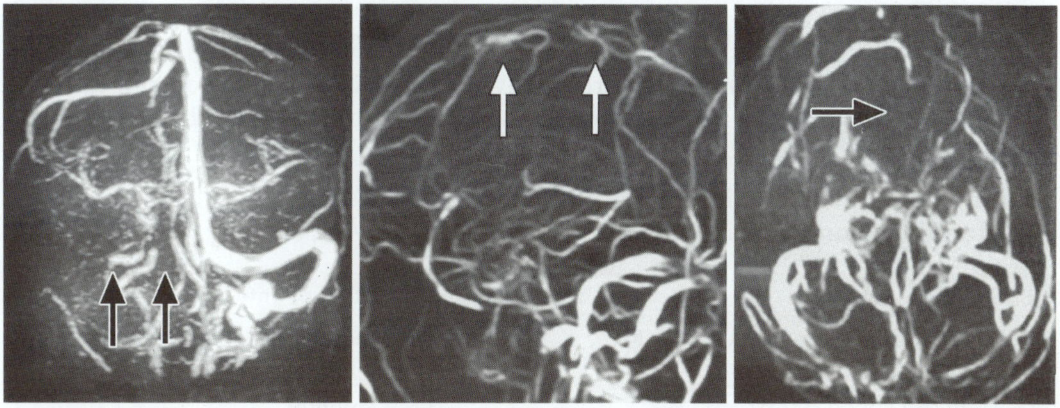

Fig. 17.3: Absence of flow on MRV

Laboratory tests

- Complete blood count, chemistry panel, prothrombin time, and activated partial thromboplastin time.
- D-dimer: Negative predictive value. Normal D-dimer level may rule out CVT.

TREATMENT

- Antithrombotic therapy
- Reversing the underlying cause when known
- Control of seizures
- Control of intracranial hypertension

EARLY ANTICOAGULATION

- Early anticoagulation with either subcutaneous LMWH or intravenous UFH

- LMWH is preferred unless the patient is planned for an invasive procedure (lumbar puncture, decompressive craniotomy), when UFH can be given and stopped before procedure.
- *The presence of hemorrhagic venous infarction, intracerebral or isolated subarachnoid hemorrhages are **not** contraindications for anticoagulation.*

Anticoagulant	Dose
Unfractionated heparin	80 U/kg iv bolus followed infusion at 18 U/kg/hr
Low molecular weight heparin	• Enoxaparin: 1 mg/kg q12 h • Dalteparin: 200 U/kg q24 h or 100 U/kg q12 h • Fondaparinux: ◆ <50 kg–5 mg q24 h ◆ 50–100 kg–7.5 mg q24 h ◆ >100 kg–10 mg q24 h

LONG-TERM ANTICOAGULATION

- Shift to oral anticoagulants like warfarin/NOACs after initial parenteral anticoagulation.
- The dose of warfarin should be titrated to maintain an INR of 2–3.

Endovascular treatment: In case of progressive neurologic worsening despite adequate anticoagulation, endovascular thrombolysis or mechanical thrombectomy can be attempted.

Duration of anticoagulation:

The duration of anticoagulation depends on the underlying etiology of CVT:

Etiology	Duration of anticoagulation
Provoked CVT by a transient risk factor (ex: pregnancy, drugs, trauma)	3–6 months
Unprovoked CVT	6–12 months
Recurrent CVT, CVT with thrombophilia like APLA	Lifelong

SUPPORTIVE THERAPY

Raised intracranial pressure

1. Elevate head end
2. Osmotic therapy (mannitol or hypertonic saline)
3. Hyperventilation to maintain pCO_2
4. Hemicraniectomy in severe cases with impending herniation

Seizure prophylaxis

- For patients with seizures/supratentorial lesions on neuroimaging.
- Levetiracetam: 20 mg/kg loading dose followed by 1 gm twice daily which can be increased up to 1.5 gm twice daily.

Infection and inflammation

- CNS infection and local infection (mastoiditis, sinusitis)—treat with IV antibiotics.
- IV glucocorticoids are indicated if underlying etiology is of inflammatory origin.

Chapter

18

Status Epilepticus

Neurological emergency: It is important to stop seizure activity before neuronal loss.

Definition: The International League Against Epilepsy (ILAE)

Status epilepticus as 'a single epileptic seizure of greater than ***30 minutes*** duration or a series of epileptic seizures during which function is not regained between ictal events in a 30 minute period'.

Period of 30 minutes is not practical, hence a functional definition of 5 minutes duration is kept to initiate the treatment.

Classification

1. **Convulsive status epilepticus**
   a. Generalised status epilepticus
   b. Focal onset evolving into generalised status epilepticus
   c. Myoclonic status epilepticus
   d. Focal motor status epilepticus
2. **Non-convulsive status epilepticus**
   a. Non-convulsive status epilepticus with coma
   b. Non-convulsive status epilepticus without coma
      - Absence status epilepticus
      - Focal status epilepticus without impairment of consciousness
      - Focal status epilepticus with impaired consciousness

Etiology

1. Anti-seizure drug nonadherence in patients with prior epilepsy
2. Acute structural brain injury (e.g. stroke, head trauma, subarachnoid hemorrhage, cerebral anoxia or hypoxia), infection (encephalitis, meningitis, abscess), or brain tumor.
3. Remote/long standing injury (e.g. prior head injury or neurosurgery, arteriovenous malformations, and benign brain tumors)
4. Withdrawal syndromes from alcohol, barbiturates, or benzodiazepines
5. Metabolic abnormalities (e.g. hypoglycemia, hepatic encephalopathy, uremia, hyponatremia, hyperglycemia, hypocalcemia and hypomagnesemia).

6. Drugs that lower the seizure threshold (e.g. theophylline, quinolones, imipenem, high-dose penicillin G, cefepime, metronidazole, isoniazid, tricyclic antidepressants, bupropion, lithium, clozapine, lidocaine, bupivacaine).

DIAGNOSIS

- Clinically obvious status epilepticus must be treated immediately and there is no need for EEG.
- A neurological examination is important in making the diagnosis of subtle or focal forms of status epilepticus.
- No alteration of consciousness, asymmetric features, and automatic movements may indicate a focal lesion.
- Continuous EEG is necessary for the diagnosis of non-convulsive status epilepticus.
- Rule of thumb: Generalized seizures (bilateral movements always cause loss of consciousness).

MANAGEMENT

Rapid assessment and support

1. A rapid neurologic examination for etiology.
2. Airway, breathing, and circulation: Supportive therapy (e.g. oxygen, mechanical ventilation) should be instituted.
3. Blood drawn for electrolytes including calcium, sodium, phosphorus, and magnesium, serum glucose, liver function tests, a complete blood count, toxicology studies, and anti-seizure drug levels, as appropriate.
4. GRBS to be done: Thiamine (100 mg) and dextrose (50 ml of 50% dextrose solution) should be given, if hypoglycemia is present.

Pharmacological Therapy

Impending and Early Status (5–30 mins)

1. First-line treatment:

Benzodiazepines

- *Lorazepam*
  - 0.1 mg/kg IV at a maximum rate of 2 mg/minute.
  - Repeat after 3–5 minutes, if the patient continues to seize.
  - There is no maximum dose.
- *Diazepam* 0.15 mg/kg IV, up to 10 mg per dose as second choice
- If IV access is not available, give *midazolam* 10 mg IM stat.

To prevent further seizures

- Fosphenytoin infusion of 20 mg/kg phenytoin equivalents (PE) should be started at 100–150 mg/min

  1 PE fosphenytoin = 1 mg phenytoin sodium = 1.5 mg fosphenytoin sodium, or Phenytoin infusion of 20 mg/kg infusion in normal saline at 25–50 mg/min.

The infusion rate should be reduced if significant adverse effects occur.

If seizures persist:

- An additional dose of 5–10 mg PE/kg fosphenytoin/phenytoin can be given 10 minutes later, up to a maximum cumulative dose of 30 mg/kg.

Note

Phenytoin (but not fosphenytoin) is incompatible with benzodiazepines/dextrose. Hence two IV access should be obtained)

Alternatives to phenytoin and fosphenytoin

1. **Valproate:** Loading dose of 30 mg/kg followed by infusion at 10 mg/kg/min. Maximum dose 3 gm, or
2. **Levetiracetam:** 40–60 mg/kg IV can be given over 15 minutes, or
   3 gm administered as an infusion at a rate of 2 mg/kg/min, or
3. Lacosamide 400 mg IV stat, followed by 200 mg IV 12th hourly, especially in partial onset seizures

   Any metabolic abnormality found should be promptly corrected.

Refractory Status Epilepticus

Ongoing convulsive or nonconvulsive seizures even after administration of an initial benzodiazepine/non-benzodiazepine anti-seizure drug, given in appropriate doses.

Refractory status epilepticus may be divided into two phases:

1. Early (3 min to 48 hours)
2. Late (>48 hours)

Continuous EEG monitoring should be instituted as soon as possible, along with continuous pulse oximetry and blood pressure monitoring, often with an arterial catheter.

Management

1. Continue all antiepileptic drugs already started
2. Start anesthetics (in order of choice)
   A. Midazolam 0.2 mg/kg IV bolus, which can be repeated every 5–10 minutes up to 2 mg/kg total and start infusion 0.1 mg/kg/h, or
   B. Propofol 2 mg/kg IV bolus, repeated up to a maximum total dose of 10 mg/kg and infusion at 20 μg/kg/minute, or
   C. Pentobarbital 5 mg/kg IV loading dose over 10 mins, followed by infusion at 1 mg/kg/h and titrate up to 5 mg/kg/h
   D. Thiopental 4 mg/kg IV loading dose and 0.3–0.4 mg/kg/min infusion
3. Continue anesthetics for 24–48 hours after seizure control

Super-refractory Status Epilepticus

If none of the above measures control the seizures, use general anesthesia, and this is labeled as super-refractory status epilepticus.

The anaesthetic agents which can be used include: Isoflurane, desflurane, ketamine.

Other therapies include:

1. Topiramate 300–1600 mg/d via gastric tube.
2. Magnesium 4 g bolus IV and 2–6 g/h infusion (keep serum levels <5 mg/dL). Dilute in 12 ml saline and give over 5–20 minutes.

3. Pyridoxine 100–600 mg/d IV or via gastric tube.
4. Ketogenic diet: 4:1—Fat: Carbohydrates, protein diet.
5. Immunomodulator agents like:
   A. IVIg 0.4 g/kg/d IV for 5 days
   B. Plasma exchange for 5 sessions
   C. Methylprednisolone 1 gm/day for 5 days followed by oral prednisone 1 mg/kg/day for 1 week
6. Neurosurgical consultation for resection of epileptogenic focus.
7. New modalities: Vagal nerve stimulation, deep brain stimulation, repetitive transcranial magnetic stimulation.

Post-ictal period: Investigate for cause

- A head CT/MRI should be obtained once seizures are controlled.
- A lumbar puncture (LP) for acute infections of the central nervous system.

Usage of anti-convulsants in status epilepticus in renal and hepatic dysfunction:

Drug	Renal modification	Hepatic modification
Phenytoin	No dose modification	No dose modification
Fosphenytoin	No dose modification	No dose modification
Valproate	No dose modification	Contraindicated in hepatic dysfunction
Midazolam	No dose modification However, in patients receiving continuous infusion cannot adequately eliminate the metabolites, hence can lead to prolonged sedation despite stopping.	No dose modification
Phenobarbital	CrCl >10—no dose modification CrCl <10—dose to be given every 12–16 hr Hemodialysis—additional 50% of dose post-HD	No dose modification
Levetiracetam	According to CrCl 80–130 = 1.5 gm q12 h 50–80 = 500 mg–1 gm q12 h 30–50 = 250–750 mg q12 h 15–30 = 250–500 mg q12 h <15 = 250–500 mg q24 h HD- 500–1 gm every q24 h post HD (or) If prior dose given then an additional dose of 250–500 mg to be given post-HD	No dose modification
Lacosamide	Based on CrCl >30—no dose modification <30—reduce to 75% of the maximum dose HD—75% of the max dose followed by 4 hours post-HD additional dose of 50% to be given	No dose modification

Chapter

19

Acute Bacterial Meningitis

Meningitis is the inflammation of leptomeninges and is characterised by increased white blood cells in the cerebrospinal fluid (CSF).

ETIOLOGY

Age	Common organism
Neonate (<1 month)	• *Escherichia coli* • Group B Streptococcus • *Listeria monocytogenes* • Gram-negative bacilli
Children	• *Streptococcus pneumoniae* • *Neisseria meningitidis* • *Haemophilus influenzae*
Adults (18–50 years)	• *Streptococcus pneumoniae* • *Neisseria meningitidis*
Adults >50 years	• *Streptococcus pneumoniae* • *Neisseria meningitidis* • *Listeria monocytogenes* • Gram-negative bacilli
Following invasive neurosurgical procedures—post shunting	• *Staphylococcus aureus* • Coagulase—negative staphylococci

Predisposing Clinical Situations

- **CSOM:** Pneumococcus
- **Nasal source:** Meningococcus
- **Adults >55 years and adults of any age with alcoholism or other debilitating disease:** *Streptococcus pneumoniae*, Gram-negative bacilli.
- **Hospital-acquired meningitis, post-traumatic or post-neurosurgery, immunosuppressed patients:** *Staphylococcus aureus*, *Streptococcus pneumoniae*, Gram-negative bacilli.

Clinical features of acute bacterial meningitis

- Fever (>80%)
- Headache (>85%)
- Neck rigidity (>80%)
- Nausea and vomiting (~35%)

Due to meningoencephalitis

- Altered consciousness (>75%)
- Seizures (30%)
- Focal neurological signs (10–35%)

The classic triad of fever, headache and neck rigidity may be present in only about 40%.

Signs

- Kernig's sign: Pain on full extension of the knee when the hip is flexed 90°.
- Brudzinski's sign: Spontaneous flexion of the hips during passive flexion of the neck. Both signs have a low sensitivity–5% and a high specificity–95%

Initial Approach

- For any suspected case of meningitis **treatment should be started within an hour of diagnosis**.
- Blood cultures should be immediately taken and started on empirical therapy.
- CSF examination by lumbar puncture to be done as soon as possible and sent for investigation.

Neuroimaging (by CT/MRI) is **not mandatory** prior to lumbar puncture but is needed in patients with:

a. Focal neurological deficit
b. Papilledema
c. New onset seizure
d. Immunocompromised state
e. Prior history of CNS disease (mass, stroke)

CSF Findings in meningitis	Bacterial	Viral	Partially treated bacterial
CSF opening pressure	Raised	Raised	Normal
WBCs	500–10000/µl	25–500/µl	100–1000/µl
RBCs	Absent	Absent	Absent
Glucose	Very low <40 mg/dL (CSF: Serum ratio 0.4)	Normal	Normal
Protein	Very high (>200 mg/dL)	20–80 mg/dL	>45 mg/dL
Gram stain	Positive in 60%	Negative	Negative
Culture	Positive in 80%	Viral PCR positive	Negative

TREATMENT

Empirical Antimicrobial Therapy

- Patients with suspected bacterial meningitis should be started on antibiotic therapy along with dexamethasone.
- Empiric antibiotics
    - Adults <50 years: Ceftriaxone 2 g IV q12 h plus vancomycin 15–20 mg/kg IV q8–12 h
    - Adults ≥50 years or immunocompromised: Ceftriaxone 2 g IV q12 h plus vancomycin 15–20 mg/kg IV q8–12 h plus ampicillin 2 g IV q4 h

Targeted Antibiotics (always given IV)

Duration of therapy: Depends on the underlying organism and generally given for 7–10 days.

1. Meningococcus for at least 7 days
2. Pneumococcus and Staphylococcus for at least 14 days
3. Pseudomonas/GNB for 21 days

Repeat Lumbar puncture needed only if

1. No improvement after 48hours of initiation of antibiotics
2. 48–72 hours after initiation of antibiotics in pathogens like penicillin resistant Pneumococcus, Gram-negative bacilli (health care associated)

Streptococcus pneumoniae, Neisseria meningitidis	
Penicillin–sensitive	• Penicillin G 20–24 million units/day, given in divided doses every q4 hourly (or) • Ampicillin 2 gm every q4 hourly
Penicillin-resistant	• Ceftriaxone 2 gm every q12 hourly (or) • Cefotaxime 2 gm every q4 hourly (or) • Cefepime 2 gm every q8 hourly • Vancomycin in Pneumococcus 15 to 20 mg/kg IV every 8 to 12 hours
Gram-negative bacilli	
Gram-negative bacilli (except pseudomonas)	• Ceftriaxone 2 gm every q12 hourly (or) • Cefotaxime 2 gm every q4 hourly
P. aeruginosa	• Ceftazidime 2 gm every q8 hourly (or) • Cefepime 2 gm every q8 hourly (or) • Meropenem 2 gm every q8 hourly
Staphylococcus	
Methicillin-sensitive (MSSA)	• Oxacillin or nafcillin 2 g IV q4 hourly (or) • Ampicillin 2 gm every q4 hourly
Methicillin-resistant (MRSA)	Vancomycin 15 to 20 mg/kg IV every 8 to 12 hours
Other organisms	
Listeria monocytogenes	Ampicillin 2 gm every q4 hourly + gentamicin 7 mg/kg/day given in three divided doses
H. influenzae	• Ceftriaxone 2 gm every q12 hourly (or) • Cefotaxime 2 gm every q4 hourly (or) • Cefepime 2 gm every q8 hourly
Acinetobacter	Meropenem 2 gm every q8 hourly

SUPPORTIVE THERAPY

1. Dexamethasone: IV 0.15 mg/kg IV 6th hourly should be administered 20 minutes prior to initiation of antibiotics. Continued for 4 days.
2. Treat ICT (refer to Chapter 15: CVA)
3. Manage seizures with anti-epileptic medications
4. Care of unconscious patient (refer to Chapter 23: Coma)

Prognosis

- Mortality rate is 3–7% in meningitis caused by *Neisseria meningitidis, Haemophilus influenzae* or group B streptococci,
- 15% for *Listeria monocytogenes* and 20% for *Streptococcus pneumoniae.*

BRAIN ABSCESS

- Surgery
  - Aspiration and drainage of the abscess under stereotactic guidance.
  - Complete excision is reserved for multiloculated abscesses or when stereotactic aspiration is unsuccessful.
- Empirical antibiotic therapy for brain abscess.

Source	Antibiotic
Oral, otogenic, sinus	• Metronidazole 500 mg IV q8 hourly **plus** • Ceftriaxone 2 gm IV q12 hourly (or) • Cefotaxime 2 gm IV q4 hourly
Haematogenous spread	Vancomycin 15 to 20 mg/kg IV 8 to 12 hours
Postoperative neurosurgical patients/trauma	• Vancomycin 15 to 20 mg/kg IV 8 to 12 hours **plus** • Ceftazidime 2 gm every q8 hourly (or) • Meropenem 2 gm every q8 hourly (or) • Cefepime 2 gm every q8 hourly

- Subsequent antibiotics should be based on culture and sensitivity.
- Duration: Minimum 6–8 weeks—IV antibiotics
- Anticonvulsant therapy—continued for at least 3 months after resolution of the abscess.

VIRAL MENINGOENCEPHALITIS

Etiology

1. Enteroviruses
2. Herpes simplex ($HSV_2 > HSV_1$)
3. Japanese encephalitis
4. Varicella zoster (VZV)
5. Dengue
6. Chikungunya
7. Influenza
8. Measles
9. Cytomegalovirus (CMV)
10. Epstein-Barr virus (EBV)

Clinical Features

- Fever
- Altered or depressed level of consciousness
- Focal neurological symptoms
- Seizures

- Symptoms and signs of meningeal irritation (photophobia and nuchal rigidity) are usually absent with a pure encephalitis, but often accompany meningoencephalitis.

Diagnostic Tests

- CSF analysis
- Neuroimaging—MRI
- EEG

CSF Analysis

- Increased WBC, 250–500 cells/mm^3. Predominant lymphocytes.
- >1000 suggest a non-viral cause, however certain viruses like mumps, EEE virus, California virus and LCMV can have this type of investigations.
- Atypical lymphocytes may be seen in EBV, CMV, HSV.
- Hemorrhagic (>500 RBCs): Hemorrhagic encephalitis of HSV.
- Elevated protein concentration, but usually <150 mg/dL.
- Usually normal glucose concentration (>50 percent of blood value), but moderately reduced values are occasionally seen with HSV, mumps, or some enteroviruses.
- CSF PCR can prove the following viruses:

  a. HSV
  b. EBV
  c. CMV
  d. HHV-6
  e. Enteroviruses
  f. VZV

Neuroimaging: MRI patterns in viral meningoencephalitis

- HSV encephalitis: Increased T2-weighted signal in bilateral temporal lobes.
- Varicella-zoster virus: Multiple areas of infarction in both hemispheres.
- West Nile virus encephalitis increased signal on flair MRI of the basal ganglia
- Enterovirus encephalitis: increased signal intensity on flair MRI in both hemispheres, more in the posterior cerebral hemisphere.
- JE is characterized by grey matter involvement, whereas Nipah virus encephalitis is associated with multiple, small, white matter lesions.

EEG

1. The most common abnormality is generalized slowing.
2. Focal EEG abnormalities, especially temporal lobes, in 75 to 80% of patients with HSV encephalitis.
3. Common abnormalities: Frontotemporal slowing, temporal sharp or spike activity, and periodic lateralizing epileptiform discharges (PLEDs) at a rate of 2 to 3 Hz.

Diagnosis is made by a combination of clinical, radiological, virological and MRI criteria.

MANAGEMENT

- Primarily symptomatic and includes use of analgesics, antipyretics, and antiemetics.
- Anti-convulsants.

DEFINITIVE TREATMENT

- Acyclovir: In case of HSV-1, 2, VZV, EBV—10 mg/kg IV q8 hourly. (Total dose: 30 mg/kg/day) for 5–7 days which is **followed by**.
- Oral administration as acyclovir (800 mg five times daily), famciclovir (500 mg Tid) or valacyclovir (1 gm Tid) for a total course of 7–14 days
- There is no specific therapy of proven benefit for arboviral encephalitis.

Renal dose modification of acyclovir

CrCl	Dose
CrCl >50	No dosage adjustment necessary.
CrCl 25 to 50	10 mg/kg/dose every 12 hours
CrCl 10–25	10 mg/kg/dose every 24 hours
CrCl <10	5 mg/kg/dose every 24 hours
Intermittent hemodialysis (IHD)	2.5 to 5 mg/kg/dose every 24 hours. Administer after hemodialysis on dialysis days
Continuous renal replacement therapy (CRRT)	5 to 10 mg/kg/dose every 24 hours

Chapter

20

Guillain-Barré Syndrome

Guillain-Barré syndrome (GBS) is an acute, frequently severe, and fulminant polyradiculoneuropathy that is autoimmune in nature.

Variants of GBS

- Acute inflammatory demyelinating polyneuropathy (AIDP)
- Acute motor axonal neuropathy (AMAN)
- Acute motor and sensory axonal neuropathy (AMSAN)
- Miller-Fisher
- Pharyngeal-cervical-brachial weakness
- Bickerstaff encephalitis
- Acute pandysautonomia
- Pure sensory GBS
- Paraparetic variant

CLINICAL FEATURES

1. Progressive, **symmetrical proximal weakness** of the legs and arms, ranging from minimal weakness to complete paralysis of all four limbs, bulbar and facial muscles.
2. **Areflexia** or decreased reflexes in the limbs.
3. Weakness usually sets in **within hours to days** and progresses over **days to four weeks** with the **nadir of symptoms at 2 weeks**.
4. Cranial nerve involvement, bifacial nerve palsy, and bulbar palsy.
5. Mild sensory symptoms tingling dysesthesias in the extremities (80%), mild loss of pain and temperature sensation (AMSAN variant).
6. Autonomic disturbances (in 20 to 70%): Fluctuations in blood pressure, postural hypotension and cardiac dysrhythmias.
7. Antecedent events: 70% of cases of GBS occur **1–3 weeks after an acute infectious** respiratory or gastrointestinal, like *Campylobacter jejuni*, Epstein-Barr virus, cytomegalovirus, HIV, hepatitis E, Zika, *Mycoplasma pneumoniae*, COVID-19.

   The following features make the diagnosis of **GBS less likely**:

   - Sensory level/severe sensory signs with little or no muscle weakness at onset
   - Bowel and bladder dysfunction at onset, or persistent, severe dysfunction.

- Severe respiratory dysfunction with little or no limb weakness at onset.
- Fever at the onset of weakness/Marked, persistent asymmetry of weakness.

DIFFERENTIAL DIAGNOSIS

1. **Periodic paralysis (hypo- and hyperkalemia)**—must be ruled out in all cases.
2. Metabolic myopathies (hypokalemic, hyperkalemic).
3. HIV vacuolar myelopathy.
4. Tick paralysis.

INVESTIGATIONS

Nerve conduction studies:

- Demyelinating forms of GBS—conduction blocks.
- Axonal forms of GBS—decreased motor and/or sensory amplitudes.

Cerebrospinal fluid analysis: Albuminocytologic dissociation.

- Elevated CSF protein (100–1000 mg/dL) with normal CSF white blood cell count (<5 cells/mm^3).
- A transient increase in white cell count (5–50 cells/mm^3) may be present in about 15% cases.
- LP done within one week can be normal. Better to do after that.

Antibodies

Variants	IgG autoantibodies to
AIDP	GM1 (<50%)
AMAN	GM1, GD1a
AMSAN	GM1, GD1a
Pharyngeal-cervical-brachial	GT1a > Gq1b >> GD1a
Miller Fisher	Gq1b, GT1a
Bickerstaff encephalitis	Gq1b, GT1a

Laboratory testing for antibodies other than Gq1b is not performed routinely in view of limited clinical utility.

MRI

Only if needed to rule out other differentials.

DIAGNOSTIC CRITERIA (BRIGHTON CRITERIA)

- **Clinical features:** Bilateral and flaccid weakness of limbs + decreased or absent tendon reflexes + monophasic illness pattern and interval between onset and nadir of weakness between 12 hours and 28 days and subsequent plateau
- **Electrophysiologic studies:** Nerve conduction studies consistent with GBS
- **CSF:** Cytoalbuminologic dissociation

MANAGEMENT

Definitive Treatment

- Plasma exchange (plasmapheresis).
- Intravenous immunoglobulin (IVIG).
- Both are equally efficacious.

Indications

- Non-ambulatory patients with GBS within 4 weeks of symptom onset.
- Ambulatory GBS not recovering within 4 weeks of symptom onset.

Patients who are mildly affected and already recovering do not require disease-modifying therapy.

Intravenous Immunoglobulin (IVIG)

Total dose of 2 gm/kg weight administered over 5 days (0.4 gm/kg/day)

How to administer

1. Prior to initiation of IVIG infusion, ensure normal volume status
2. **Infusion rate:** 0.01–0.02 mL/kg/min, for the first 30 minutes preferably using an infusion pump; increase to maximum 0.06 mL/kg/min, if no adverse reactions are observed.
3. Avoid rapid IV infusion in patients with renal dysfunction/thrombotic risk
4. If an adverse reaction occurs during IVIG infusion, decrease the rate of infusion or stop the infusion until the reaction subsides.

   The most common **adverse reactions (≥5%)**
   - Flu like symptoms: Headache/asthenia (fatigue)/pyrexia
   - Anaphylaxis/acute renal failure
   - MI/CVA, DVT, pulmonary embolism

Plasmapheresis

A course of 40–50 mL/kg plasma exchange 4–5 times over 7–10 days.

Venous access: Requires reliable vascular access, two large, durable peripheral veins or a central dual-lumen. Radiographic confirmation of catheter placement.

Fluid volume removed by apheresis must be replaced by:

- 5% albumin,
- Saline (for hyperviscosity)
- Combination of albumin and saline

Complications of plasmapheresis

1. Hypotension
2. Hypersensitivity reactions
3. Edema

SUPPORTIVE MANAGEMENT

Respiratory Failure

Parameters predicting a high risk of respiratory failure

- Time of onset, to admission with respiratory failure <7 days.
- Inability to cough vigorously
- Inability to stand
- Inability to lift elbows and abduct shoulder
- Inability to lift head

In patients with at least four of these, mechanical ventilation was required in >85 percent of patients.

Indication for intubation

- Worsening weakness of neck muscles, upper limbs, increased respiratory distress.
- **Single Breath Count:** <20, suggests respiratory weakness (normal: 40–50)
- PFT parameters (Mnemonic: 20–30–40)
  - FVC <20 mL/kg
  - Maximum inspiratory pressure (MIP) <30 cm H_2O
  - Maximum expiratory pressure (MEP) <40 cm H_2O
- Ventilation till the patient is cured by definite treatments.

Autonomic dysfunction

- **Arrhythmias:** Atrial and ventricular arrhythmias and conduction blocks.
- Treat on its own merit

Blood pressure: Paroxysmal hypertension and orthostatic hypotension.

- Intra-arterial BP for severe fluctuations in blood pressure.
- Hypotension should be treated with fluids.
- Episodes of severe hypertension (MAP >125 mm Hg) can be treated with labetalol, esmolol or nitroprusside.

Bowel and bladder: Urinary retention and paralytic ileus possible, hence daily abdominal auscultation for bowel sounds is recommended.

DVT prophylaxis: For immobility.

Chapter

21

Myasthenic Crisis

Myasthenic crisis is a life-threatening condition that is defined as worsening of myasthenic weakness requiring intubation or noninvasive ventilation.

Precipitants

A. Concurrent infections/surgery

B. Pregnancy and postpartum period

C. Medications

1. Antibiotics: **Aminoglycosides**/fluoroquinolones/sulfonamides/penicillins/nitrofurantoin
2. Magnesium containing medications (e.g. laxatives, antacids)
3. Cardiovascular medications: Beta-blockers/calcium channel blockers
4. Neuromuscular blockers (e.g. succinylcholine)

DIAGNOSIS

Clinical

- Ptosis, dysphagia, dysphonia
- Respiratory distress assessed by single breath count: Normal is 40/min
- Inability to complete sentences in one breath, paradoxical breathing, etc.

On ventilator

- VC (vital capacity) falls below 15 to 20 mL/kg
- MIP (mean inspiratory pressure) is less negative than –25 to –30 cm H_2O (i.e. between 0 and –30 cm H_2O)
- If above features present, consider intubation and ventilation

Differential diagnosis: **Cholinergic crisis**

- Cholinergic crisis is rare in patients on pyridostigmine <120 mg every 3 hours.

  Hence even in the presence of cholinergic side effects, the worsening muscular weakness should be attributed to myasthenia and treated accordingly.

	Myasthenic crisis	Cholinergic crisis
Heart rate	Tachycardia	Bradycardia
Pupil	Normal/dilated	Constricted
Secretions	Normal	Increased secretions
Skin	Faint and cold	Warm and flushed
Tensilon/edrophonium test	Improves weakness	Detrimental

TESTS FOR MYASTHENIA

Edrophonium Test: Historical importance—not done routinely

Neostigmine Challenge Test

- Neostigmine: 1.5 mg IM or 0.5 mg IV
- Preloaded with atropine 0.6 mg to prevent muscarinic side effects.
- Improvement of ptosis following neostigmine observed

Ice Pack Test

- Simple bedside test, high specificity (96%) and sensitivity (82%) for myasthenia
- An ice pack is applied to the weak eyelid for 5 minutes, ensuring that the ice is covered to prevent ice burns, and an improvement of palpebral fissure of at least 2 mm is considered a positive test.

Electrophysiological Tests

- Rapid reduction in the amplitude of compound muscle action potentials (CMAP) >10% during repetitive stimulations of a peripheral nerve
- Reversal of this response by neostigmine or edrophonium
- Single-fiber electromyography (EMG): More sensitive method of detecting the defect in neuromuscular transmission.

MANAGEMENT

General Principles

Supportive care

- Admit to intensive care unit
- Consider elective intubation if:
  - Signs of respiratory distress/respiratory acidosis/plenty of oral secretions
- Stop anticholinesterase drugs in intubated patients to avoid excess airway secretions
- Treat precipitating or contributing factors, particularly infections

Definitive treatment

- The main therapies for myasthenic crisis are plasma exchange and IVIG.
- These start to work within several days, but the benefits last only a few weeks.
- For details, refer to Chapter 20: Gullian-Barré Syndrome.

Plasma exchange

- Dose: Five exchanges (3 to 5 L of plasma each) over 7 to 14 days.
- Plasma exchange done on alternate days is effective in reducing the antibody levels.
- Patient shows improvement usually after the second or third exchange.

IVIG therapy

- The dose of IVIG is 2 g/kg, over 2 to 5 days (e.g. 400 mg/kg per day over 5 days)
- Improvement occurs in a few days and up to 2 weeks and usually lasts weeks to months.

Immunomodulation therapy

Prednisolone 1 mg/kg for longer benefit, as plasma exchange and IVIG is short lived.

Note: There may be transient worsening of weakness 5–10 days after initiating steroids (in up to 50%) and may worsen respiratory function to require intubation (in 10%), and last 5–6 days. However, this transient worsening may be prevented if the patient is undergoing plasma exchange or IVIG treatment.

Long-term immunosuppressant

- Mycophenolate mofetil: In adults 2 to 3 g/d divided in 2 doses given 12 hourly.
- Azathioprine: Therapeutic dose is 2 to 3 mg/kg/day.

The therapeutic effect takes 4 to 8 months with azathioprine and a few weeks to 2 months with mycophenolate mofetil.

Anticholinergic treatment

- Restart pyridostigmine after recovery from crisis.
- Starting dose: Pyridostigmine 30 mg three times a day 30 minutes before meals (maximum dose is 120 mg every four hours).
- Effect starts in 30 to 60 minutes and lasts for 3 to 4 hours.
- Every 4 hours while the patient is awake if diplopia is the main symptom.

Weaning from ventilatory support

- Consider extubation when the patient is clinically better, and has better ventilatory parameters and ABG.

Chapter

22

Delirium

DEFINITION

Delirium: Acute state of altered consciousness characterized by disordered attention, with diminished speed, clarity, and coherence of thought.

Predisposing factors

- Age ≥65 years
- Comorbid illnesses
- Impaired cognition, vision and hearing
- Alcohol misuse
- Depression/past history of delirium
- Admission in hospital, especially ICU with loss of circadian signals

ETIOLOGY

1. Metabolic disorders—encephalopathy
    - Electrolyte abnormalities: Sodium, calcium, glucose/hypoxia/hypercapnia
    - Uremia/hepatic encephalopathy/thiamine and B_{12} deficiency
    - Endocrinopathy: Hypothyroidism/hyperthyroidism/adrenal insufficiency
2. Infectious illness
    - Septic encephalopathy (underlying source being pneumonia/CNS infections/urosepsis/peritonitis/endocarditis, etc.)
3. Drugs and medications
    - Opiates/barbiturates/serotonergic antidepressants
    - Cannabinoids/dopaminergic agonists
    - Corticosteroids/anticholinergics
    - Alcohol
4. CNS disorders
    - Hypertensive encephalopathy
    - Focal ischemic strokes and hemorrhages/subdural hematoma
    - Nonconvulsive status epilepticus/post-ictal states
    - CNS vasculitis/neurologic paraneoplastic/autoimmune encephalitis
5. Neoplastic disorders
    - Secondary metastasis/primary CNS tumors/carcinomatous meningitis

EVALUATION

Identify: Clinical tool

Confusion Assessment Method (CAM)

A. Acute onset and/or fluctuating course
B. Inattention
C. Disorganized thinking (irrelevant talk, unclear flow of ideas)
D. Altered consciousness (alert, vigilant, lethargic, stupor, coma)

Diagnosis is made by the presence of A and B with either C or D.

HISTORY

Most of the history in the patients are usually obtained from a relative or a bystander. The history should be aimed at identifying an underlying cause.

The key points to establish from history include:

- Baseline cognitive function
- The time course of the disease
- Medication history—over the counter/herbals, including any recent change in dose or substitution of medication

PHYSICAL EXAMINATION

The initial examination should be focussed and include:

1. Vitals
2. Assess the level of consciousness/neurological examination
3. Screening for signs of underlying etiologies

INVESTIGATIONS

1. Appropriate work up for all encephalopathies based on etiology
    - Complete blood picture/serum electrolytes/renal function tests (uremic encephalopathy)/liver function tests (hepatic encephalopathy)
    - Arterial blood gas analysis (hypoxia/hypercapnia/acid-base status)
2. Screening for systemic infection: Chest X-ray/urinalysis/blood culture
3. Neuroimaging:
    - Non-contrast CT: Look for hemorrhage, ischemic stroke, mass lesions
    - MRI-brain: Acute ischemic stroke, and anatomical details regarding infectious/inflammatory/neoplastic lesions.
4. Lumbar puncture: In patients with suspected CNS infections should be obtained after neuroimaging.
5. Electroencephalogram (EEG): To exclude seizure especially non-convulsive seizure
6. Serum and drug toxicology screening.
7. Other tests:
    - Thyroid function tests, serum cortisol levels, B_{12}, thiamine levels.
    - Autoimmune serology: Antinuclear antibodies (ANA), complement levels; p-ANCA, c-ANCA and paraneoplastic/autoimmune encephalitis serologies.

- Infectious serologies: Rapid plasmin reagin (RPR); fungal and viral serologies if high suspicion; HIV antibody.

TREATMENT

- Treatment of the underlying etiology
- Supportive care

Supportive care

- Reassurance, touch, and verbal orientation can lessen disruptive behaviors.
- A well-lit room with activities or exercises during the day and a quiet, dark environment with limited interruptions during night is important in an ICU as constant activity can provoke delirium.
- Reorientation by the nursing staff and family combined with visible clocks, calendars, and outside-facing windows can reduce confusion, especially in ICU.
- Proper nutrition and volume status as well as managing pain, and proper skin care.
- Sensory isolation should be prevented by providing glasses and hearing aids to patients who need them.
- Managing agitation
  A. Haloperidol: Low dose (0.5–1 mg) with maximum of 5 mg/day. Given—orally, IM, or IV onset of action—5 to 20 minutes after IV.
  B. Quetiapine 50 mg once daily (titrated up to 100 mg every 24 hours) up to a maximum dose of 400 mg/day, may reduce delirium duration.
  C. Lorazepam (0.5–1 mg): Primarily used in alcohol withdrawal. Can be increased up to 2 mg tid in this context.
  D. Dexmedetomidine infusion may reduce rate of delirium in mechanically ventilated patients available—200 μg/2 mL
    - Loading: 1 μg/kg IV over 10 minutes;
    - Maintenance 0.2–0.7 μg/kg/hr continuous IV infusion
  E. Physical restraints should be a last resort as they can cause problems, such as loss of mobility, pressure ulcers, and prolonged delirium.

Chapter

23

Coma

Coma is a state of impaired responsiveness, in which the patient is in a deep sleep-like state with eyes closed from which they cannot be aroused.

It differs from the vegetative state, in which a person is awake, with eyes open, but does not have any meaningful response to stimuli.

Causes

I. Structural

Vascular

- CVA-infarction—large infarct in anterior and posterior circulation
- Intracerebral bleed/subarachnoid hemorrhage/hypertensive encephalopathy
- Subdural/epidural bleed
- Cerebral vasculitis

Nonvascular

- Head trauma—contusion and concussion
- Post-ictal state
- Non-convulsive status epilepticus
- Heat stroke
- Hydrocephalus

ICSOL

- Cerebral abscess
- Tuberculoma/toxoplasmosis
- Metastasis to brain

II. Non-structural

Metabolic

- Hypoxia/hypercapnia
- Hypoglycemia/hyperglycemia—HHS, DKA
- Hypernatremia/hyponatremia
- Hypocalcemia/hypercalcemia
- Hypothermia/hyperthermia

- Hepatic encephalopathy
- Uremic encephalopathy
- Hypothyroidism—myxedema coma

Infections and parainfectious

- Bacterial meningitis
- Viral encephalitis
- Postinfectious encephalomyelitis/acute demyelinating encephalomyelitis
- Tropical illnesses—cerebral malaria, scrub typhus, leptospirosis, enteric fever
- Bacterial infections in elderly: Pneumonia/UTI

Toxins/drugs

- Alcohol
- OP poisoning
- Sedatives, hypnotics, anti-psychotics, tranquilizers
- Carbon monoxide, cyanide, methanol, ethylene glycol

Others

- Diffuse cerebral ischemia (postcardiac arrest, heart failure, arrhythmia)
- Myocardial infarction

History

- Onset of symptoms—acute, subacute, fluctuating
- History of fever
- Preceding seizures, focal neurological deficits, head trauma,
- History of raised intracranial pressure—early morning headache, projectile vomiting
- History of drug/toxin exposure

Past history: COPD/bronchial asthma/cirrhosis/CKD/epilepsy/diabetes/hypertension/IHD.

- **Habits:** Alcoholism/smoking/drug addiction
- **Drug history:** Diuretics/OHAs/insulin

Examination

- Assess vitals first:
  - Pulse rate
    - Bradycardia—raised intracranial pressure
    - AF—embolic stroke
- Hypertension
    - CVA—IC bleed or thrombosis
    - If very high—PRES, hypertensive encephalopathy
- Hypotension—shock-sepsis, cardiac failure, Addison's crisis
- Carotid artery bruit—for evidence of narrowing, in stroke patients
- Hypo-/hyperthermia—both a cause and an effect secondary to impaired hypothalamic function
- Breathing pattern
  - Hypo-/hyperventilation
  - Abnormal patterns of breathing—due to brainstem injury during transtentorial herniation, Cheyne-Stokes, ataxic, apneustic breathing

- Cyanosis—for hypoxia and hypercarbia
- To look for systemic involvement—polycythemia, purpura, lymph nodes, edema, eschar, subconjunctival bleeds, signs of liver cell disease, renal failure, etc.

Anemia	Blood loss, hematological malignancies chronic kidney disease, alcoholism
Cyanosis	COPD, asthma
Clubbing	Bronchogenic carcinoma, cirrhosis of liver
Edema	Cardiac failure, renal failure, cirrhosis of liver
Lymphadenopathy	HIV, tuberculosis, lymphoma
Jaundice	Hepatic encephalopathy, cirrhosis of liver
Bleeding/purpura	Hematological malignancies, septicemia, leptospirosis
Skin rashes/blisters	Vasculitis, meningococcemia, barbiturate poisoning
Fever	Meningitis, encephalitis, cerebral malaria, enteric fever Septicemia
Hypothermia	Myxedema coma, chronic kidney disease
Hypertension	Cerebrovascular accident, SAH, hypertensive encephalopathy
Hypotension	Shock
Dehydration	Electrolyte imbalance, shock-hypovolemic/septic
Smell of poison	Poisoning

- Facial trauma, with raccoon eyes, bruising of mastoids (battle sign)—can be suggestive of underlying facial and skull bone fracture with possibility of IC bleed/traumatic brain injury

Neurological Examination

- Assess level of consciousness

Glasgow Coma Scale

Eye opening	Spontaneous	4
	Response to verbal command	3
	Response to pain	2
	No eye opening	1
Best verbal response	Oriented	5
	Confused	4
	Inappropriate words	3
	Incomprehensible sounds	2
	No verbal response	1
Best motor response	Obeys commands	6
	Localizes pain	5
	Withdrawal response to pain	4
	Flexion to pain	3
	Extension to pain	2
	No motor response	1
≥13—mild brain injury; 9–12—moderate brain injury; ≤8—severe brain injury		

- Posturing: Usually a structural brain lesion; can also happen in deep metabolic coma
  Decorticate
  - Upper-extremity adduction and flexion at the elbows, wrists, and fingers
  - Lower-extremity extension
  - Lesion-bilateral damage rostral to the midbrain

  Decerebrate
  - Upper-extremity extension, adduction, and pronation
  - Lower-extremity extension
  - Lesion-damage to motor tracts caudal to the midbrain
- Multifocal myoclonus—metabolic/toxic injury; hypoxic ischemic encephalopathy
- Fundus: For papilloedema, HTN/DM/SAH
- Pupils:
  1. Pin-point pupils—pontine hemorrhage/lesions (due to decreased sympathetic outflow)/opioid overdose/OP poisoning
  2. **Asymmetrical pupils**
     a. Unilateral dilated pupil
        i. Due to 3rd nerve/nucleus injury;
        ii. False localising sign, due to transtentorial herniation
     b. Horner's syndrome—miosis on one side
  3. Fixed dilated pupils—transtentorial/brainstem herniation
- Eye movement
  - Doll's eye—oculocephalic manoeuvre—lost in severe brainstem lesions and in profound toxic/metabolic insults—never to be elicited in patients with possible head or neck trauma.
  - The presence of a doll's eye in a comatose patient shows that the brain stem is still intact.
- Eye position
  - May indicate brainstem strokes
  - Caloric test can also be used
- Conjugate deviation of the eyeballs is toward the affected side in destructive lesions of the frontal lobe, and away from the affected side in irritative lesions.
- Corneal reflex: Absent if brainstem is affected.
- 6th nerve palsy: False localising sign for ICT/pontine lesion.
- Facial nerve: UMN palsy in strokes above pons; LMN palsy—in pons.
- 9th, 10th—in strokes above medulla transiently, and in Wallenberg's syndrome.
- **Most important**: Look for focal neurological deficit—paucity of movements of one side (when given a central painful stimulus, like sternal pressure), hypo-/hypertonia, asymmetrical DTRS, upgoing plantar.

  Note: Generally focal deficits point to a structural lesion in the brain.
  Rarely, hypoglycemia can present with hemiplegia, as an exception.
- Signs of meningeal irritation
- RS: For aspiration pneumonia
- CVS: For heart disease causing embolic stroke
- Abdomen: Liver and spleen

Investigations

Three important parameters to be recorded: ***Blood sugar*** to be done first in all to rule out hypoglycemia, ***oxygen saturation*** for hypoxia and ***blood pressure*** for hypotension/ hypertension.

Blood tests

- Complete blood picture
- Liver and renal function tests
- Arterial blood gas analysis
- Serum electrolytes—sodium, potassium, calcium, magnesium
- Thyroid function tests
- Serum ammonia
- Blood culture/work up for tropical illness (malaria/leptospirosis/scrub typhus/ dengue)
- HIV screening
- Toxin screen

Neuro-imaging

CT to be done first, followed by MRI based on requirement

  - CT—to look for gross structural lesions, especially IC bleeds and ICSOLs; negative for infarction in first 6 hours
  - MRI—superior for identifying ischemic stroke, CNS infections, characterising the ICSOL. For hypoxic encephalopathy, do MRI after 72 hours

- Lumbar puncture and CSF analysis—to look for infections, SAH, malignant cytology
- Electroencephalogram (EEG)—primarily for diagnosing non-convulsive status epilepticus
- Carotid—vertebral Doppler for strokes

Cardiac workup

- ECG—for AF, IHD, MI, chamber hypertrophy
- ECHO—for EF, wall motion abnormalities.

Differential Diagnosis (Table 23.1)

Table 23.1: Disorders of consciousness

	Awareness	Wakefulness	Brain stem/ respiratory	Motor	EEG	Prognosis
Brain death	Absent	Absent	Absent	Absent	Electro-cerebral silence	Brain dead: Heart and respiration will cease soon. Can be considered for organ donation

Contd.

Table 23.1: Disorders of consciousness (Contd.)

	Awareness	Wakefulness	Brain stem/ respiratory	Motor	EEG	Prognosis
Coma	Absent	Absent	Depressed, variable	Reflex or posturing	Polymorphic delta, burst suppression	Variable-based on cause
Vegetative state	Absent	Present, intact sleep-wake cycles	Intact	Reflex, non-purposeful	Delta, theta, or electro-cerebral silence	Poor, when chronic
Minimally conscious state	Intact but poorly responsive	Intact	Intact	Variable with purposeful movements	Nonspecific slowing	Variable
Locked-in syndrome	Intact but communication difficult	Intact	Intact breathing; often brain stem signs	Quadriplegia, pseudobulbar palsy	Usually normal	Poor

Management

- Secure A, B, C
- *Airway and breathing:* If GCS is less than 8, to intubate to protect airway, except in post ictal states where consciousness is likely to return soon
- Check GRBS and correct hypoglycaemia with 50 mL of 50% dextrose IV stat. Thiamine is given along with dextrose to prevent Wernicke's encephalopathy.
- Oxygen supplementation if hypoxic
- If MAP <70 mm Hg (shock)—IV fluids and inotropes
- If MAP >130 mm Hg: Appropriate anti-hypertensive therapy if it is a hemorrhage
- *Rewarming:* If hypothermia is present
- Empirical antibiotic therapy after lumbar puncture, if sepsis is a likely cause of coma
- Treat underlying cause—electrolyte imbalance, raised ICT, infection, etc.

Supportive Care in an Unconscious Patient

- After initial management
- Pass a Ryle's tube; stomach wash if poisoning or GI bleed is suspected
- Connect condom catheter drainage if incontinent
- Catheterise the bladder if urinary retention is present
- Nutrition and hydration
  - Start RT feeding at the earliest—if there are no contraindications, as IV fluids alone will not provide all the sufficient calories and nutrients. Use 20–30 calories/kg and 1 gm/kg protein.
  - Monitor intake and output of the patient and accordingly adjust input the next day

  - Electrolytes and renal functions to be monitored as required
  - Salt, vitamins, minerals and trace elements—supplementation to be given
- Care of the eyes—to prevent exposure keratitis
  - Neosporin eye ointment and eye shields to keep eyes close
- Care of the back to prevent bedsores
  - Frequent change of position (2nd hourly)
  - To keep skin dry by using talcum powder
  - Avoid folds in the bed sheet
  - Nurse on a water/air bed
- Chest physiotherapy and intermittent throat suction to clear secretions
- Maintain oral hygiene by washing/suction
- Head end elevation at 30–45 degrees/lateral position to avoid aspiration
- IV pantaprozole 40 mg od for ulcer prophylaxis
- DVT prophylaxis–mechanical stockings or UFH 5000 IU 12th hourly/enoxaparin 1 mg/kg od subcutaneously
- Care of the endotracheal tube—periodic sterile suctioning and ideally periodic transient cuff deflation
- Care of the IV access
  - Look for evidence of infection
  - Always follow aseptic precautions
  - Change once in 2–3 days or if there is evidence of cellulitis or thrombophlebitis.

Section

3

Pulmonary

Chapter

24

Acute Severe Asthma

Clinical Features

History

- Most adult patients will have a history of prior asthma or use of bronchodilators.
- Classic symptoms include:
  - Wheeze (high-pitched whistling sound, usually upon exhalation)
  - Cough (often worse at night)
  - Shortness of breath or difficulty breathing
  - Chest tightness
- Episodic symptoms
- History of exposure to particular triggers such as allergens, infections.
- History of other allergic conditions, e.g. atopic dermatitis, allergic rhinitis

Examination

- Tachycardia >120 bpm, RR >30/minute
- Blood pressure: Hypotension <90 mm of systolic
- Pulsus paradoxus in severe asthma
- Cyanosis in severe asthma
- Tachypnea
- Dyspnea: Use of accessory respiratory muscles
- Inability to complete sentences
- On auscultation—bilateral polyphonic expiratory rhonchi
- In very severe asthma there might be absent breath sounds due to severe bronchoconstriction—silent chest.

Investigations

Saturation by probe <94%

- Arterial blood gas analysis
  - Mild or moderate asthma—type 1 respiratory failure and hypoxia
  - Severe asthma—type 2 respiratory failure, due to severe bronchoconstriction, causing CO_2 retention or even normal CO_2.

- Chest X-ray to look for:
  - Pneumonia that could have triggered the acute exacerbation of asthma
  - Pneumothorax—close differential diagnosis for silent chest/due to asthma
- PEFR <50% predicted

Differential Diagnosis

- Acute exacerbation of COPD (previous history, older age group, smoker)
- Cardiac asthma or acute pulmonary edema (patient with IHD or hypertension, older age, first time wheezing)
- Foreign body obstruction (children)
- Eosinophilic pneumonia with systemic vasculitis—Churg-Strauss syndrome (rare)

Treatment

- Supplemental oxygen should be started to ensure SpO_2 >92%
- Bronchodilators are the mainstay of treatment and they include:
  - Nebulized short acting B_2 agonists (SABA)—which include:
    - Levosalbutamol 2.5 to 5 mg every 20 minutes for 3 doses, then every 1 to 4 hours as needed, or 10 to 15 mg/hour continuously.
    - Onset of action—15 minutes
    - Stacked inhalations of multi-dose inhalers (MDI) (salbutamol) can be done at home, before reaching emergency, if patient is trained well on MDI use
  - Nebulized anticholinergics
    - Ipratropium—500 μg every 20 minutes for 3 doses, repeated every 4 hours
  - Nebulized steroids—such as:
    - Budesonide—given as 400 μg stat and then 4th hourly
    - Others include—beclomethasone, fluticasone, etc.
  - IV glucocorticoids—will take 4–6 hours for onset of action
    - IV methylprednisolone 60 to 80 mg stat and 6–12 hours for patients in ICU. Can be given as 40 to 60 mg IV 12 to 24 hours non-intensive care
    - IV hydrocortisone 200 mg IV stat, with 100 mg IV 8th hourly is alternative regimen
  - IV magnesium sulphate: In refractory bronchoconstriction
    - Inj magnesium sulphate 2 g IV given over 20 minutes diluted in normal saline stat single dose.
    - Contraindicated in renal insufficiency
- **Indications for intubation and ventilation:**
  - Decreased respiratory rate,
  - Altered mental status or drowsiness
  - To decrease respiratory effort if patient is tiring
  - Oxygen saturation <92 percent even with high-flow supplemental oxygen
  - Type 2 respiratory failure with severe hypoxia. ***A normal CO_2 may also be dangerous and indicate respiratory muscle fatigue.***
- NIV can be tried for a few hours, if the patient is conscious and cooperative.

- Antibiotics indicated only if:
  - History of an infection (fever, increased counts, CXR suggestive of pneumonia)

Nonstandard therapies:

  - Slow infusion of theophyllines: Loading dose—4–6 mg/kg
    - Maintenance—0.3 to 0.4 mg/kg/hour (500 mg in 500 mL dextrose to run at 15–30 mL per hour)
    - Should be used with caution with patients with underlying cardiac condition due to risk of arrhythmias. It can also precipitate convulsions.
  - Inj terbutaline 0.25 mg SC stat 8th hourly (caution-elderly, cardiac problems)
  - Inj adrenaline 0.5 mg SC stat and every 20 min for 3 doses (caution as in terbutaline)
  - At discharge: Counsel patient to do stacked MDIs if recurrence of acute attacks.

Chapter

25 Acute Exacerbation of Chronic Obstructive Pulmonary Disease (COPD)

Global initiative for chronic obstructive lung disease (GOLD) defines an exacerbation of COPD as **an acute event characterized by a worsening of the patient's respiratory symptoms** that is beyond normal day-to-day variations and leads to a change in medication.

Acute change of cardinal symptoms:
1. Cough increases in frequency and severity
2. Dyspnea increases in severity
3. Sputum production increases in volume and/or changes character

Triggers for the exacerbations include:
- Bacterial infections (>50%)—*Strep. pneumoniae, Haemophilus influenzae, Moraxella catarrhalis, Mycoplasma pneumoniae, Chlamydia pneumoniae*
- Viral infections (30%)—H_1N_1, coronavirus.
- Nonspecific triggers in the remaining cases

Clinical Examination

- Inability to complete sentences
- Respiratory rate >30/min
- Heart rate >120/min
- Cyanosis/hypoxia (<90% saturation on room air)
- Use of accessory muscles of respiration
- Bilateral extensive rhonchi: If severe bronchoconstriction, very high pitched rhonchi, silent chest
- Bronchial breathing and crepitations for pneumonia
- CO_2 narcosis—drowsiness, ***asterixis***
- Right heart failure/pulmonary HTN—raised JVP, pedal edema, parasternal heave, loud P_2.

Investigations

- Arterial blood gas analysis—hypoxia/hypercarbia (COPD patients may have chronic compensated respiratory acidosis; pCO_2 high, HCO_3 high, pH normal.)
- CXR: For consolidation/pneumothorax
- Complete blood count, blood glucose, renal function tests, serum electrolytes,

- ECG—look for arrhythmias (MAT), cor pulmonale, lead I sign of emphysema
- Echocardiogram—for cor pulmonale and rule out IHD
- CRP: May be used to guide antibiotic therapy
- Blood culture/sputum culture/throat swab for influenza as needed
- Trop T, NT proBNP: If cardiac cause suspected

Treatment

- **Oxygen:** Lowest percentage of oxygen should be started to target SpO_2 of 88 to 92%. Use nasal oxygen, then venturi (28–60%).

  Higher saturation can cause hypercapnia due to reduced respiratory drive. (COPD patients depend on hypoxia for the respiratory drive. If this is removed, they may not breathe adequately).
- **Noninvasive ventilation (NIV)**
  - Indications:
    - Persistent hypoxia despite supplemental oxygen therapy (if patient is conscious and cooperative and BP is normal)
    - Increased work of breathing/signs of respiratory muscle fatigue
    - Respiratory acidosis (pH $\leq$7.35) and/or hypercapnia (pCO_2 $\geq$45 mm Hg)
- Use non-invasive positive pressure ventilation, with IPAP (inspiratory positive airway pressure) of 8–12 mm Hg and EPAP (expiratory positive airway pressure) of 5 mm Hg adjusted to deliver adequate minute ventilation.
- Trial only for 2–4 hours
- **Indications for intubation and ventilation:**
  - Severely impaired consciousness,
  - Inability to clear secretions or protect airway
  - Poor respiratory effort/fatigue
  - Severe hypoxia (PaO_2 < 60 mm of Hg), pH < 7.25.
  - Higher than normal pCO_2 is common in COPD patients, and not an indication if there is no acidosis, or drowsiness.
  - Hypotension
  - When NIV has failed or contraindicated
- Bronchodilators
  - Beta agonists—Levosalbutamol—1.25 to 2.5 mg every 20 minutes for 3 doses, then 1.25–5 mg every 1 to 4 hours as needed via nebulizers
  - Anticholinergic agent: Ipratropium 500 micrograms via nebulizer stat and 6th hourly
  - Glucocorticoids—very useful. Decrease hospital stay, hastens recovery and reduce future relapses, especially if the patient is already on low dose steroids.
    - Onset of action, after 4 hours
    - IV methylprednisolone 40–60 mg stat and 6th hourly. Can be used up to 125 mg 6th hourly also.
    - Replaced by prednisolone 40 mg daily for 5 to 14 days when better.

- *Theophyllines*: Its role is controversial. It may not be useful, can cause arrhythmias, convulsions and hypotension if given IV. If used, must be done with caution, in the lowest dose.
- *Mucolytics:* Not proven to be effective. Patients should be encouraged to cough and clear secretions. Hot fluids are good mucolytics
- Antimicrobials
  - Empirical antibiotics–
  - For LRTI:
    - Inj amoxicillin clavulanate 1.2 g IV q8 h
    - Inj azithromycin 500 mg q24 h
  - For pneumonia or extensive lung involvement with hypotension:
    - Inj piperacillin tazobactam 4.5g IV q8 h
  - Antibiotics can be changed based on the culture sensitivity
  - Duration of antibiotics: 5–7 days
  - Antivirals—if suspecting viral etiology
    - Oseltamivir 75 mg bd × 5–10 days
- Right heart failure—cor pulmonale:
  - Oxygen—preferred therapy
  - Frusemide —20 to 40 mg IV and then titrated as per urine output
  - Digoxin—0.125 to 0.25 mg daily
  - Sildenafil—20 mg daily tid, can be increased to 80 mg tid
  - Thromboprophylaxis (mechanical or pharmacological) if in ICU

Note

If patient does not improve as expected, look for:
- Small undetected pneumothorax
- Resistant/untreated respiratory infection.
- Pulmonary embolism.

Chapter

26

Tension Pneumothorax

Life-threatening condition, where air is trapped in pleural cavity by a one way valve, causing air to enter and not leave the pleural space.

Aetiology

- COPD—emphysema, rupture of emphysematous bullae
- Acute severe asthma
- Rupture of cavity in lung-pneumatocele—*Staph.aureus* (usually pyopneumothorax)
- Bronchogenic carcinoma (usually hemopneumothorax)
- Blunt trauma
- Iatrogenic:
  - Barotrauma
  - Procedures: Central venous catheter insertion, chest drain insertion

Symptoms

- Acute onset dyspnea
- Chest pain (pleuritic type)

Signs

- Increased respiratory rate/tachycardia
- Pulsus paradoxus
- Cyanosis
- Hypotension

Respiratory System

- Accessory muscle use
- Decreased chest movements on the affected side
- Gross tracheal and mediastinal deviation to the opposite side
- Hyper-resonant percussion note
- Decreased breath sounds/absent tactile/vocal fremitus
- Subcutaneous emphysema may be present, especially in traumatic and advanced cases

Recognition in Mechanically Ventilated Patients

- Worsening hypoxia
- Increasing peak airway pressures

Differential Diagnosis

- Acute pulmonary embolism
- Myocardial infarction
- Pneumonia

Chest X-ray Findings

- Contralateral shift of trachea and mediastinum
- Absent bronchovascular markings on affected side
- Collapsed lung border may be visualised on side of pneumothorax

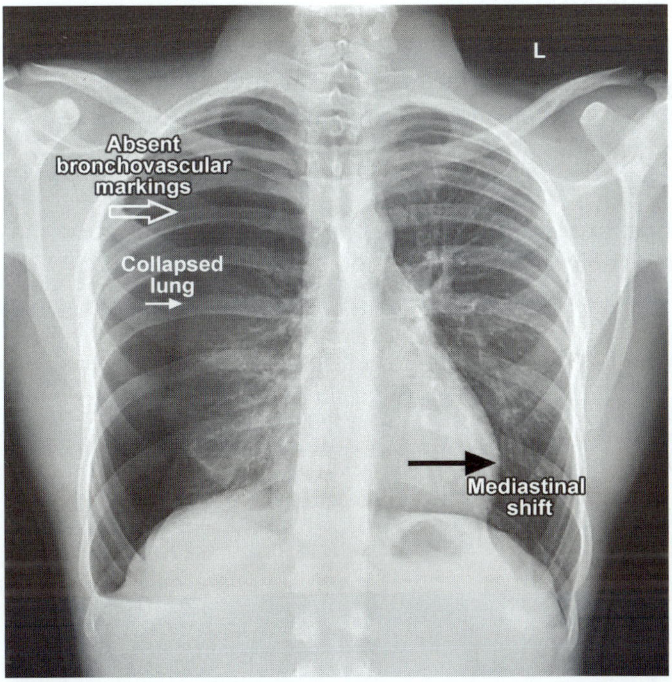

Fig. 26.1: Chest X-ray showing right sided pneumothorax: Collapsed right lung border, absent lung markings on right side, and mediastinal shift to opposite side

ABG

- Hypoxia and hypercarbia

Ultrasound Findings

- Absence of lung sliding/absence of lung pulse/presence of lung point.

MANAGEMENT

1. Patients are usually hemodynamically unstable and require immediate intervention.
2. Start oxygen at 60% venturi. Can increase to 100%. It also helps reabsorption of nitrogen in pleural space.

3. If ultrasound is available, bedside scan to confirm the diagnosis of pneumothorax should be done.
4. If ultrasound is unavailable, chest X-ray can be done.
5. Do not wait for confirmatory imaging and based on clinical assessment decisions to intervene should be taken.
6. Needle decompression using a wide-bore needle (temporary measure): Done as an emergency measure to release air, as we prepare for intercostal drainage Use a wide bore needle and syringe and draw air from pleural cavity .
7. Intercostal tube insertion: Most definitive, life saving treatment

   Intercostal tube drain should be inserted in the fourth or fifth intercostal space in the mid-axillary line or 2nd space anteriorly connected to an underwater seal and fixed.
8. Intubation and mechanical ventilation
   - For persistent hypoxia
   - Use lower tidal volumes and low positive end expiratory pressures (PEEP)
   - Should be done only after placement of an intercostal drainage tube
9. The drain can be removed the day after the lung has been fully re-expanded (on CXR) and the bubbling has been stopped in the drain (shows bronchopleural fistula has closed).

   If bubbling stops, but the lung is not expanded, then the tube may be blocked, or kinked, or out of the pleural space. Reposition it.

Note

Avoid clamping the ICD if patient is breathless.

Chapter

27

Massive Hemoptysis

DEFINITION

Blood loss of 400 mL in 24 hours or 100–150 mL expectorated at one time

Common Causes

- Cavitary tuberculosis (TB)/post-TB bronchiectasis
- Basal bronchiectasis
- Pulmonary embolism
- Bronchogenic carcinoma/adenoma
- Lung abscess
- Aspergilloma
- Bleeding diathesis

Treatment of Hemoptysis

1. Airway and breathing
    - Clear airway
    - Intubation if the patient is unable to protect the airway or is hypoxic and requires ventilation
    - Oxygen supplementation, mechanical ventilation
    - Place patient in lateral decubitus with bleeding site down if source of bleeding known
2. Circulation: Assess hemodynamic stability:
    - Check BP, look for orthostatic hypotension
    - Blood transfusion: If patient is hypotensive and Hb is low
    - Crystalloids: If hypotensive, without drop in Hb. Give IV fluid NS or RL at 100–200 mL/hr, based on age, cardiac and renal status. Monitor urine output.
3. Rule out pseudohemoptysis (from upper airway) and hematemesis.
4. Investigations: Must be carried out simultaneously to find cause
    - Rule out bleeding tendencies: BT, CT, PT and platelet counts
    - CBP and appropriate cultures to rule out infection.
    - Chest X-ray—to look for obvious evidence of TB, bronchogenic carcinoma, bronchiectasis, lung abscess.

CT Scan Thorax

- If CXR is normal, always do a contrast enhanced CT scan of the thorax, which may pick up the site of bleeding, and identify all the four above mentioned causes.
- CT pulmonary angiography—for diagnosis of pulmonary embolism

5. Bronchoscopy: It is done
   i. To identify the site of bleeding,
   ii. Removal of blood and thrombus,
   iii. For biopsy of endobronchial lesion,
   iv. To control bleeding

- Adjuncts to bronchoscopy to assist with bleeding control include
   i. Lavage with cold saline
   ii. Topical medications (e.g. epinephrine)
   iii. Balloon tamponade
   iv. Local thermal ablative procedures

6. Reversal of coagulopathy with antifibrinolytic agent—inhaled tranexamic acid 500 mg (using injectable solution) 3 times daily for up to 5 days, may be tried.
7. Additional measures to protect non-bleeding lung such as single lung ventilation or double-lumen endotracheal tubes may be required in patients in whom life-threatening bleeding continues despite initial measures
8. If no further active bleeding: Conservative therapy
   - Most mild to moderate hemoptysis will settle in 24 hours:
   - Sedatives and anxiolytics, e.g. lorazepam 1 mg bd
   - Cough suppressants like codeine may help
   - Treat infection with broad spectrum antibiotics, as it is the commonest precipitating cause for hemoptysis.
   - Inj hemocoagulase(botropace) 1 amp IV/IM 8th hourly can be tried .
9. If bleeding persists:
   - Embolization of bleeding vessel can be done after identifying by angiography in a tertiary care center
   - Success rate depends on identifying the artery and subsequent embolization, and may vary from 50 to 90%.
10. Further refractory bleeding: Surgery (usually lobectomy)
   - For patients who fail bronchoscopic or arteriographic interventions
   - Early surgery may be indicated in:
     - Chest trauma
     - Iatrogenic pulmonary artery rupture
     - Refractory bleeding from an aspergilloma
     - Bronchovascular fistula

Chapter

28

Pneumonia

DEFINITION

Pneumonia is defined as the infection of the pulmonary parenchyma. Classified as –

- Community-acquired pneumonia (CAP)
- Hospital-acquired pneumonia (HAP) that occurs ≥48 hours after admission,
- Ventilator associated pneumonia (VAP)—pneumonia which occurs >48 hours of ventilation.
- Healthcare-associated pneumonia—cases of CAP that are caused by multidrug-resistant (MDR) pathogens typically associated with HAP.

Clinical Features

Symptoms

1. High-grade fever with chills and rigors
2. Cough with or without sputum production
3. Dyspnea—if extensive involvement
4. Chest pain (pleural involvement—20–30%)
5. Atypical organisms like Legionella present with GI symptoms such as nausea, vomiting, or diarrhea
6. Others—altered sensorium–septic encephalopathy/Legionella

Signs

If pneumonia is large: Tachycardia/tachypnea/hypoxia/hypotension

Chest Findings

- Decreased chest movements/dull note on percussion
- Tubular bronchial breath sounds/increased vocal resonance, aegophony
- Crepitations/pleural rub/effusion

COMMUNITY-ACQUIRED PNEUMONIA

Etiology

Typical organisms	Atypical organisms
Streptococcus pneumoniae *Haemophilus influenzae* *Klebsiella pneumoniae* *Pseudomonas aeruginosa* *Staphylococcus aureus*	*Mycoplasma pneumoniae* *Chlamydia pneumoniae* Legionella Respiratory viruses—influenza A and B, rhinovirus, respiratory syncytial virus, coronavirus

Epidemiologic Factors Suggesting a cause of CAP

Factor	Organism
Alcoholism	*Streptococcus pneumoniae* ***Klebsiella pneumonia*/Anaerobes**
COPD and/or smoking	***Haemophilus influenzae/Streptococcus pneumoniae*** *Pseudomonas aeruginosa* Legionella/Moraxella/*Chlamydia pneumoniae*
Structural lung disease (bronchiectasis)	***Pseudomonas aeruginosa*** *Staphylococcus aureus/Burkholderia cepacia*
Dementia, stroke, decreased consciousness causing aspiration	**Oral anaerobes** Gram-negative bacteria
Lung abscess	Klebsiella/MRSA/oral anaerobes
HIV	*S. pneumoniae/H. influenzae* *M. tuberculosis/Pneumocystis jiroveci*
Exposure to air conditioning	*Legionella pneumoniae*
Exposure to bats	*Histoplasma capsulatum*
Exposure to birds	*Chlamydia pneumoniae*
Exposure to rabbits	*Francisella tularensis*
Exposure to sheep, goats, cats	*Coxiella burnetii*

DIAGNOSIS

Radiology

Chest X-ray may show:

- Lobar consolidation with air bronchogram—specific not sensitive.
- Infiltrates/pneumonitis
- Synpneumonic effusion

Lab Investigations

Initial investigations sent are-

1. ABG—if patient is hypoxic-type 1 respiratory failure
2. Complete blood picture (increased TLC with neutrophilia)
3. Sputum culture and sensitivity

4. Blood culture
5. Urinary antigen—*S. pneumoniae* and Legionella
6. Nasopharyngeal/throat swab for influenza virus/COVID-19
7. Biomarkers—CRP, procalcitonin are increased
8. Multi-organ dysfunction: RFT/LFT deranged

Management

Severity of illness scores help guide whether to hospitalize the patient. Each point is one score.

CURB-65 Criteria

- Confusion
- BUN ≥20 mg/dL/urea > 40 mg/dL
- Respiratory rate ≥30/min
- Blood pressure (SBP <90/DBP <60 mm Hg)
- Age ≥ to 65 years
- Score of 0–1—outpatient treatment
- Score of 2—admission to medical ward
- Score of 3 or higher—admission to intensive care unit (ICU)

Treatment

General Measures

1. Treat septic shock if present with IV fluids and inotropes (refer to septic shock)
2. If patient is hypoxic start O_2 supplementation (refer to ARDS)
3. If hypoxia further worsens: Mechanical ventilation

Initial Antibiotic Treatment

Inpatients ICU
A. Respiratory fluoroquinolone (moxifloxacin 400 mg od , or Levofloxacin 750 mg IV od) or B. A beta lactam plus a macrolide • Ceftriaxone 2 gm IV od or ampicillin 1 to 2 gm IV q4 h–q6 h or cefotaxime 2 gm IV q8 h plus • Azithromycin 1 gm IV followed by 500 mg od or clarithromycin 500 mg oral bd
Special considerations
If Pseudomonas • Piperacillin/tazobactam (4.5 g IV q8 h), cefepime (2 g IV q8 h), imipenem (500 mg IV q6 h), meropenem (1 g IV q8 h) The above β-lactams **plus** an aminoglycoside-amikacin (15 mg/kg qd) **plus** azithromycin • The above β-lactams plus an aminoglycoside plus an antipneumococcal fluoroquinolone either ciprofloxacin (400 mg IV q12 h) or levofloxacin (750 mg IV od) or
Community acquired MRSA: • Add linezolid (600 mg IV q12 h) or vancomycin (15 mg/kg 8h to q12 h initially, with adjusted doses) plus clindamycin (600 mg q8 h)
Influenza: • Tab oseltamivir 75 mg bd × 5–10 days

Contd.

Contd.

COVID-19 (for patients with hypoxia—Severe COVID 19)
• Inj remdesivir 200 mg IV on day 1, followed by 100 mg IV od × 5–10 days • Dexamethasone 6 mg od × 10 days for patients on supplemental oxygen/mechanical ventilation • Monoclonal antibody therapy for preventing severe disease ◆ Tocilizumab 8 mg/kg (maximum 800 mg at one time) over 1 hr. Can be repeated after 12–24 hr ◆ Casirivimab 1200 mg + imdevimab 1200 mg (regeneron) single infusion IV within 10 days of symptoms

Once the cultures/RT-PCR is available change to specific agents.

Duration of Treatment

American Thoracic Society (ATS)/Infectious Diseases Society of America (IDSA) guidelines recommend that patients with CAP should be treated for 5 days.

Switched to oral: Patients improving clinically, hemodynamically stable, and able to take oral medications.

Injectable to be switched to oral when patients are improving clinically, are hemodynamically stable, and are able to take oral medications.

Before stopping antibiotics patient should be:

1. Afebrile for 48 to 72 hours
2. Breathing without supplemental oxygen (unless required for pre-existing disease),
3. No more than one clinical instability factor (defined as heart rate >100 beats/minute, respiratory rate >24 breaths/minute, and SBP ≤90 mm Hg).

Note

If patient does not respond as expected and fever continues/hypoxia increases, look for:

- Empyema—missed easily in ICU on AP view CXRs
- Lung abscess formation
- Resistant organism/wrong choice of antibiotics
- Bronchial obstruction

In patients with MRSA pneumonia:

1. Without bacteremia: 7 days, if responding to therapy within 72 hours of treatment.
2. With bacteremia: 14 days of treatment
3. With metastatic complications of bacteremia/immunocompromised patients, longer courses (e.g. ≥4 weeks).

Chapter

29

Acute Respiratory Distress Syndrome (ARDS)

Berlin definition (diagnostic criteria):

- Onset of dyspnea within 1 week of presentation or suspected clinical insult.
- Bilateral infiltrates on CXR or CT Thorax which cannot be explained by any other pathology.
- Exclusion of pulmonary edema, i.e. absence of left atrial hypertension.
- Hypoxia as defined by the ratio of arterial oxygen tension (PaO_2) to fraction of inspired oxygen (FiO_2), that is, PaO_2/FiO_2.

  The severity of the hypoxemia correlates with the severity of the ARDS:

  These values are defined on ventilator settings that include positive end-expiratory pressure (PEEP) or continuous positive airway pressure (CPAP) ≥5 cm H_2O.
  - Mild ARDS: The PaO_2/FiO_2 ratio is >200 to ≤300,
  - Moderate ARDS: The PaO_2/FiO_2 is >100 to ≤200,
  - Severe ARDS: The PaO_2/FiO_2 is ≤100

Causes of ARDS

Direct lung injury	Indirect lung injury
Bilateral pneumonia/unilateral extensive pneumonia Aspiration pneumonia	Sepsis-due to infections: Gram-negative, Gram-positive, tropical infections (leptospirosis, dengue, scrub typhus, malaria), H_1N_1, Covid-19 , HIV related
Pulmonary contusion	Severe trauma including burns
Near drowning	Transfusion related
Toxic inhalation injury	Pancreatitis
	Drugs—amiodarone, chemotherapy drugs
	Post-CABG

The most common causes of ARDS are pneumonia, sepsis and aspiration.

*Sepsis includes all possible infective etiologies including bacterial (Gram-negative more common than Gram-negative), viral (e.g. influenza, dengue) as well as the more common tropical diseases such as leptospirosis, scrub typhus, malaria.

Pathophysiology

Can be divided into 3 phases:

1. Exudative phase
   - Lasts for 7 days after the initial insult

- Primary insult causing damage to the alveolar epithelium and the capillary endothelium. In addition, functional surfactant is lost, resulting in alveolar collapse

2. Proliferative phase
   - Lasts from day 7 to 21
   - Stage of recovery at the cellular level
3. Fibrotic phase
   - Beyond week 3 of the illness
   - These patients usually require long time oxygen, due to alveolar and interstitial fibrosis

Clinical Features

- Dyspnea/tachypnea—RR > 24
- Tachycardia
- Cyanosis—if severe
- Bilateral basal crepitations to begin with, then extensive crepitations
- Hypotension—if severe

Management

Investigations

1. ABG shows hypoxia along with respiratory alkalosis and elevated A–a gradient (suggestive of VQ mismatch). At later stages, the ABG may show hypercarbia, and respiratory acidosis, suggestive of severe ARDS, and impending respiratory arrest.
2. CXR—bilateral extensive infiltrates and atelectasis.
3. CBC—leukocytosis with left shift/leukopenia due to primary cause/sepsis
4. LFT and RFT–may be deranged secondary to shock or sepsis
5. Coagulation profile—deranged, if associated with DIC—more common in sepsis
6. ECG and ECHO—to identify cardiac cause/to rule out cardiogenic pulmonary edema.
7. Investigations to identify the inciting events—such as blood, sputum cultures, etc.

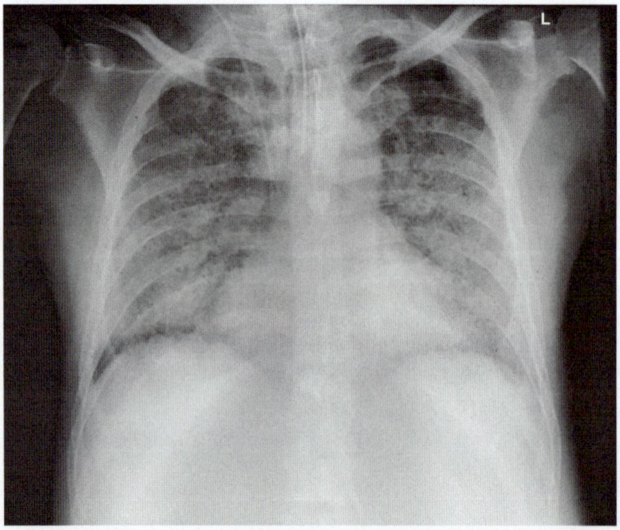

Fig. 29.1: CXR showing bilateral diffuse opacities in all zones of the lungs, typical of ARDS

Treatment

A. Hypoxia

- Supplemental oxygen
- This can be given through venturi masks, non-rebreathing masks, or as high flow nasal oxygen.

  Ventilation strategies
- Many patients with ARDS require intubation and ventilation for better oxygenation. They are kept in volume or pressure control modes.

• The goals for oxygenation (and prevention of hypercapnia) include:
  - Tidal volume set at 4–8 mL/kg of ideal body weight (to minimize ventilator induced lung injury)
  - Plateau pressure of less than 30 cm H_2O
  - Respiratory rate of less than 35
  - $FiO_2 \leq 0.6$
  - Targeting SpO_2 of 88 to 92%
  - pH >7.25
  - PEEP-12 to 15 mm (high PEEP can cause alveolar over distension, leading to barotrauma, and hemodynamic instability).

  Other strategies that have been tried include:

  Permissive hypercapnia:

  Patients who require low tidal volumes and longer inspiratory time to improve oxygenation, may have a rise in PCO_2, which can be "permitted".

The PCO_2 can be accepted, provided the pH is >7.25. If there is a lesser pH, then sodium bicarbonate can be used to correct the pH if this ventilation strategy is necessary to oxygenate the patient.

• Prone position:
  - This is done to increase alveolar recruitment, and improve the V/Q mismatch.
  - Patients should be proned early in the first 48 hours of ARDS, within first 7 days only.
  - Proning is done for 12 to 16 hours.
  - Proning cannot be done if the patient is on inotropic support.
• Alternate mode of ventilation: high frequency oscillatory ventilation has been tried
• ECMO—extracorporeal membrane oxygenation serves as a lung replacement therapy for limited periods
• Inhaled vasodilators—like nitrous oxide, prostacyclin, prostaglandin E1) selectively dilate the vessels that perfuse well-ventilated lung zones, resulting in improved oxygenation due to better ventilation/perfusion (V/Q) matching and the amelioration of pulmonary hypertension.

B. Fluid Management

Dry lung policy:

• Maintain negative fluid balance but keep MAP ≥65 mm Hg and avoid hypoperfusion.
• Diuresis is essential to improve oxygenation and lung compliance.

C. Sedation and Neuromuscular Blockade

Adequate sedation and neuromuscular blockade has shown to improve mechanical ventilation.

Sedation in ICU:

- IV fentanyl (10 mL (500 mg) in 40 mL of NS)
  Loading dose 0.5 mL to 2 mL
  Maintenance: 2.5 – 5 mL /hr. Maximum dose 10 mL/hr
- IV midazolam (1 mL = 1 mg)
  Loading 0.5 mL to 5 mL
  Maintenance: 1–8 mL hr
- IV dexmedetomidine (1 mL = 100 mg. 2 mL in 48 mL NS)
  Loading 5 mL/hr
  Maintenance: 3–10 mL hr
- IV propofol (1 mL = 10 mg. No dilution needed)
  Start at 3 mL/hr
  Maintenance: 1.8–18 mL hr
- IV midazolam + morphine infusion
  (1 mL midazolam = 1 mg+ 1mL morphine = 10 mg)
  Mix to make 1 mg of each and infuse at 1–3 ml/hr

Neuromuscular blockade:

- Atracurium (10 mg/mL)
- Loading dose—25 mg stat
- Maintenance 5 mL/hr
- Modify in renal failure

D. Glucocorticoids

Useful in Covid 19 ARDS, in which it is shown to be life saving .

- Dose : Injection dexamethasone 6 mg IV od for 5 days, or
- Inj methylprednisolone 40 mg IV bd for 5 days has been recommended
- In other causes of ARDS, trials are still on for proving its efficacy.

Chapter 30

Ventilator-associated Pneumonia (VAP)

Ventilator-associated pneumonia (VAP) is a type of hospital-acquired pneumonia (HAP) that develops after more than 48 hours of intubation and mechanical ventilation.

ETIOLOGY

Common organisms

Gram-negative and Gram-positive bacteria

- *Escherichia coli*
- *Klebsiella pneumoniae*
- *Pseudomonas aeruginosa*
- *Enterobacter* spp.
- Acinetobacter
- *Staphylococcus aureus* (MSSA/MRSA)
- *Streptococcus pneumoniae*

Risk factors for multi-drug resistant (MDR) pathogens for VAP

(Pseudomonas, other Gram-negative bacilli, and MRSA)

1. Antibiotic use within the last 90 days/≥5 days of hospitalization prior to VAP
2. Septic shock/ARDS/AKI at the time of VAP

Risk factors for MRSA include

A. Prior antibiotic therapy/hospitalization
B. Known MRSA colonization/local MRSA rate >10%/unknown)
C. Chronic hemodialysis

When to suspect?

Patients on ventilator with

- New or progressive pulmonary infiltrate on CXR/CT
- PLUS supportive clinical findings of infection.
- Confirmed by respiratory cultures growing organisms.
- The most important clue is: Deterioration in the ventilatory parameters and increase in ventilatory requirements.
  - Reduced tidal volume
  - Increased inspiratory pressures needed
  - Increased FiO_2 needed

Supportive clinical findings include–

1. New onset fever
2. Tachypnea
3. Increased or purulent secretions
4. Crepitations, bronchial breath sounds

Laboratory Investigations

1. ABG: Worsening hypoxemia and hypercarbia
2. Increasing total counts and neutrophilia

Imaging

- **Chest X-ray**

  New or progressive:
  - Lobar consolidation with air bronchogram
  - Infiltrates/pneumonitis/cavitating lesions
  - Caution: Rule out atelectasis/pulmonary embolism/pulmonary edema

  Ultrasound
  - To look for:
    - Evidence of consolidation—dynamic air bronchogram
    - Detect pleural effusion
    - Synpneumonic effusion
- **CT-Scan**
  - Useful in:
    - Patients with a normal CXR but have clinical symptoms of respiratory tract infection
    - To identify extent of lung involvement

Respiratory Cultures

Respiratory cultures should be obtained prior to the change of antibiotic therapy.

- Lower respiratory tract samples should be obtained, either invasively by bronchoscopy, or by non-invasive methods, and sent for microscopy and cultures.
- **Microscopy–**
  - The presence of abundant neutrophils is consistent with VAP and the bacterial morphology may suggest a likely pathogen (e.g. Gram-negative rods).
- Quantitative cultures –
  - VAP is considered when:
    - Endotracheal aspirates—≥1,000,000 colony forming units (cfu)/mL
    - Bronchoscopic—10,000 cfu/mL
  - These thresholds establish VAP and rule out tracheobronchial colonization .

Note

Colonisation of the respiratory tract by several organisms will happen in patients on a ventilator. Growing an organism in the endotracheal tube, does not mean infection. Infection should be supported by clinical deterioration/high total counts/worsening ABG or CXR.

Blood Cultures

Many MDR organisms in susceptible hosts can invade the blood in ICUs, and hence this is an important investigation.

TREATMENT

The difficulty in treating VAP is the selection of antibiotics and increase in MDR pathogens. Since patients are sick, antibiotics cannot wait for cultures to be seen, hence empirical therapy based on local microbiological considerations is a must.

These must be changed after the organism is identified and sensitivity is available.

Empiric therapy is indicated in:

Patients with VAP who have no known risk factors for MDR pathogens

- Treatment in a unit where ≤10 percent of gram-negative isolates are resistant to an agent being considered for monotherapy
- Treatment in a unit where ≤20 percent of *S. aureus* is resistant to methicillin

Start on one agent that has activity against Pseudomonas, other Gram-negative bacilli, and methicillin-susceptible *S. aureus* (MSSA) as monotherapy

- Piperacillin-tazobactam (4.5 g IV q 8 or 6 h)
  OR
- Cefepime (2 g IV q8 h)
  OR
- Levofloxacin (750 mg IV q24 h)

Patients with Risk Factors for MDR VAP

Start **two agents** with activity **against *P. aeruginosa*** and other Gram-negative bacilli and one agent with activity against MRSA
For Pseudomonas: two agents

ONE of the following:

Piperacillin-tazobactam 4.5 g IV q8 h or 6th hourly

- Cefepime 2 g IV q8 h
- Ceftazidime 2 g IV q8 h
- Imipenem 500 mg IV q6 h
- Meropenem 1 g IV q8 h
- Aztreonam 2 g IV q8 h

Plus one of the following:

- **Aminoglycoside**
  - Amikacin 15 to 20 mg/kg IV daily
  - Gentamicin 5 to 7 mg/kg IV daily
  - Tobramycin 5 to 7 mg/kg IV daily
- **Fluoroquinolone**
  - Ciprofloxacin 400 mg IV bd
  - Levofloxacin 750 mg IV daily

- **Polymyxins**
  - Colistin is given as 9 million units loading dose followed by maintenance dose of 4.5 million units IV every 12th hourly
  - Polymyxin B: 2.5 to 3 mg/kg/day (25,000 to 30,000 units/kg/day) IV divided in two doses.
- Inhaled colistin 1–2 million units bd/tid can be used in addition to the above.

  Plus
- **One agent with activity against MRSA**
  - Linezolid (600 mg IV q12 h) (or)
  - Vancomycin loading dose of 25—30 mg/kg followed by 15–20 mg/kg IV q8 h to q12 h (or)
  - Teicoplanin (8–12 mg/kg stat) IV stat, and same dose 8th hourly, followed by same dose od (or)
  - Tigecycline 100 mg loading dose IV followed by 50 mg q12 h. Can be used at 200 mg stat, and 100 mg IV 12th hourly in resistant cases (higher dose). Never use as single agent.

Management of MDR *Acinetobacter baumannii* Infections

- Cefoperazone—Sulbactam 3 grams IV bd
- Meropenem IV (2 gm q8 h infused over 3 hours)
- Imipenem IV (500 mg q6 h)
- Colistin: 9 million units loading dose IV followed by maintenance dose of 4.5 million units IV 12 hourly. Infuse over 1 hour
- Polymyxin B: 2.5 mg/kg/day to 3 mg/kg/day (25,000 to 30,000 units/kg/day) IV in divided doses.
- Tigecycline 100 mg loading dose IV followed by 50 mg q 12 h. Can be used at 200 mg stat, and 100 mg IV 12th hourly in resistant cases.
- Minocycline 200 mg stat IV, followed by 100 mg q12 h
- Amikacin IV 15 mg/kg qd
- Inhaled colistin 1–2 million units bd/tid as additional therapy.

Management of MDR Klebsiella/*E.coli* Infections

- Meropenem (1–2 gm q8 h)
- Ertapenem (1 gm IV q24 h)
- Imipenem (500 mg q6 h)
- Ceftazidime-avibactam 2.5 gm IV q8 h
- Polymyxin is given as 2.5 to 3 mg/kg/day (25,000 to 30,000 units/kg/day) IV divided twice.
- Fosfomycin IV 20–24 grams/day
- Plazomicin (15 mg/kg once daily) aminoglycoside for treatment of complicated urinary tract infection

Note

- If a patient has a risk factor only for MDR pathogens and local MRSA resistance rates are low (i.e. <20 percent), then empiric treatment for MRSA is not needed.
- Empiric therapy should be switched to definitive therapy based on culture-sensitivity of organisms
- Duration of therapy: Minimum of 7 days; can be extended to 10–14 days, based on patient profile, and response to therapy.

Section

4

Gastrointestinal Diseases and Liver

Chapter 31

Upper Gastrointestinal Bleeding

- Bleeding from the proximal gastrointestinal tract (proximal to ligament of Treitz)
- Presents as hematemesis or melena

Major Causes

- Gastric and duodenal ulcers/duodenitis/esophagitis
- Erosive gastritis—due to NSAIDs/antiplatelet drugs/alcohol/stress ulcers
- Varices/portal hypertensive gastropathy
- Mallory-Weiss syndrome
- Carcinoma stomach
- Angiodysplasia

Other Less Common Causes:

- Dieulafoy's lesion
- Gastric antral vascular ectasia

History

Symptoms

- Hematemesis—frank blood or coffee-brown vomitus
- Melena—black tarry stools. May continue up to 3–4 days after UG bleed
- Rarely—frank bleeding PR, if there is massive ongoing bleed
- Abdominal pain/heartburn/recurrent vomiting/weight loss-based on cause

To Find the Etiology

- History suggestive of chronic liver disease
- Chronic alcohol consumption
- NSAID abuse/antiplatelets/anticoagulants
- History of other bleeding manifestations
- To distinguish pseudo-hematemesis—bleeding from upper airway, which is swallowed and later vomited out

Signs

- Tachycardia
- Orthostatic hypotension(>10% blood volume loss)
- Supine hypotension (if massive: 30% blood volume loss)

- Tachypnea, if hypoxic
- Signs of liver cell failure: Jaundice, ascites, splenomegaly, flapping tremor
- Mass abdomen—Ca stomach
- Features of generalised bleeding—to rule out bleeding diathesis
- Per rectal examination to look for black/red staining of stools

Investigations

- CBC—anemia also look for thrombocytopenia
- Grouping and crossmatch and reserve blood products for transfusion
- PT-INR/aPTT—for underlying coagulopathy
- LFT—features of cirrhosis, A/G reversal
- RFT—may have pre-renal AKI; Urea disproportionally high, because of digestion of the blood.

Definitive Diagnosis

- Upper-GI endoscopy:
  - To assess for cause
  - For definitive procedure like banding for varices/glue for ulcers
  - Timing to be decided depending on stability of patient and need for urgent intervention

Management

Principles of therapy:

- Volume resuscitation
- Stop ongoing bleed and find cause

Supportive Therapy

- Insert two large bore IV cannula
- Monitor heart rate, blood pressure, SpO_2, urine output
- Insert a nasogastric tube—aspirate out gastric contents; stomach wash with saline. Especially in patients with cirrhosis, as the blood may reach colon and cause hepatic encephalopathy if not aspirated
- To keep the patient nil per oral
- Supplemental oxygen to be started if needed/ventilation if hypoxic

Volume Resuscitation

- To give IV hydration without delay—NS/RL 100–150 ml/hr—rate based on blood loss and hemodynamic status and patient's cardiac and renal function
- Blood product transfusion

  In case of massive on-going bleed—massive transfusion protocol—1:1:1 of PRBC, platelets and FFP

  In case of major bleed, with low Hb <7 gms/dL—2 PRBCs to be transfused and reassessed.

Note

In major bleeds, initial Hb maybe normal, but will fall over the next few hours. So repeat Hb is needed in the next 6, 12 and 24 hours.

Target Hb

- in variceal bleeding is 7 g/dL (overtransfusion > 10 g/dL can worsen bleeding)
- In peptic ulcer bleeding, target Hb is >8 g/dL.
- In IHD with ischemia, higher targets of 9–10 g/dL needed.
- Platelets: To be transfused if <50,000 cells/mm
- FFP: 10–15 ml/kg, if INR >2 in patients on anticoagulation. May need 2 to 4 units per day. Transfuse each unit (200 ml) over 30 minutes. Watch for volume overload.
- Cryoprecipitate: Dose is 1 bag per 10 kg body weight; has lesser volume per unit (50–100 ml)

Pharmacotherapy

- Pantoprazole infusion 80 mg IV stat, followed by 80 mg in 36 mL NS at 4 mL/hr (8mg/hr) to continue. Can also be given q12 hrly, instead of an infusion
- Octreotide infusion—if variceal bleeding is suspected
  50 to 100 µg IV stat, followed by 500 µg in 45 mL NS at 5 mL/hr (50 µg/hr)
- Or : Terlipressin—2 mg IV bolus over 1 minute, followed by 2 mg q6 h up to 72 hours (or)
- Somatostatin—250 µg IV bolus, followed by
- 250 µg/hour infusion for 3–5 days (5 mL in 50 mL NS at 10 mL/hr)
- Vitamin K 10 mg IV slowly over 10 minutes for patients with prolonged PT. Repeat doses if needed 8th hourly. 10 mg S/C daily doses can also be given alternatively.
- To start antibiotics (IV ceftriaxone 2 g od), in cirrhotics, especially before endoscopy.
- To start anti-encephalopathy measures, in patients with cirrhosis
- To correct coagulopathy—fresh frozen plasma/vitamin K in case of cirrhosis with prolonged PT/INR in anticoagulant induced bleeding
- Prokinetics—prior to endoscopy for better visualisation;
- Metoclopramide 10 mg IV—1 hour prior to the endoscopy

To arrest bleeding

- Upper GI endoscopy
  - Both diagnostic and can be curative
  - To be done at the earliest after volume resuscitation (within 12 hours for suspected variceal bleed and within 24 hours of other bleed)
- Variceal ligation—banding is done for esophageal varices and stops bleeding
- Argon plasma coagulation of vascular ectasia, thermal coagulation/epinephrine injection for bleeding ulcers can be attempted.
- Balloon tamponade with Sengstaken-Blakemore tube can be done, if there is a delay in endoscopy.
- Rarely might require surgical/angiographic interventions, transjugular intrahepatic portosystemic shunt (TIPS), etc. based on the cause.

To prevent rebleed:

- Propranolol—10 mg Start as od/bd and increase the dose every 7–14 days;
- Can increase up to 40–120 mg/day
  - Monitor heart rate and BP
  - Heart rate around 60/m, SBP >90 mmHg
- Nitrates (Isosorbide mononitrate) can be considered if beta-blockers are contra-indicated.

Chapter

32

Acute Pancreatitis

- Acute inflammatory process of the pancreas
- Important differential diagnosis for acute onset abdominal pain

Causes

- Gallstone/biliary sludge and microcalculi
- Alcohol
- Biliary obstruction—tumors, ascariasis, periampullary diverticula
- Hypertriglyceridemia (>1000 mg/dL)
- Hypercalcemia
- Post-ERCP
- Infections—mumps, Leptospira, Salmonella, HSV, CMV, HIV
- Drugs—Azathioprine, sulfonamides, valproic acid, ART, tetracyclines
- Trauma—blunt abdominal injuries
- Anatomical—divisum, pancreatic diverticulum,
- Hereditary—SPINK, PRSS-1, CASR, CTRC, CFTR (cystic fibrosis)
- Autoimmune

Clinical Presentation

Local symptoms and signs

- Abdominal pain
  - Epigastric and periumbilical
  - Acute—continuous boring nature and radiating to back
  - Increases with food relieved on bending forward
  - Mild discomfort to severe distress
- Nausea and vomiting
- Abdominal distention—ileus/ascites
- Epigastric tenderness—maybe diffuse
- Guarding/rigidity
- Icterus—if head is involved or in biliary obstruction
- Periumbilical (Cullen) and flank discoloration (Grey-Turner)—retroperitoneal bleeding

Laboratory Investigations

- Pancreatic enzymes: Elevated lipase and amylase (>3 times upper limit of normal)
  - Lipase
    - More sensitive (82–100%)

- Starts rising within 4–8 hours of symptom onset
- Peaks at 24 hours; lasts for 8–14 days
- Amylase: Less sensitive (67–83%); (specificity 85–98%)
  - Rises within 6–12 hours of symptom onset; returns to normal by 3–5 days
  - Can be positive in parotitis, pancreatic pseudocyst, post-ERCP, alcoholism

Note

Amylase levels may be normal in pancreatitis secondary to hypertriglyceridemia.

- Other novel enzyme markers
  - Trypsinogen activation peptide (TAP)-early elevation; can predict severity
  - Trypsinogen-2 levels-serum and urine levels
- Elevated CRP/leukocytosis
- Hemoconcentration/elevated urea
- Hypocalcemia/hyperglycemia/hypoglycemia
- Liver function tests for obstructive jaundice due to gallstones

Imaging

- Abdomen X-ray
  - Colon cut-off sign—for head of pancreas
  - Sentinel loop sign—for head of pancreas and duodenum dilatation
  - Calcification of pancreas—for acute on chronic pancreatitis
- Ultrasound abdomen—diffusely enlarged and hypoechoic pancreas
  - Gallstones, peripancreatic fluid and ascites
- CECT abdomen (preferred imaging) timing: After 3 days of symptoms
  - Differentiates between acute interstitial edematous (contrast enhancing) from necrotic pancreatitis (lacks contrast enhancement) pancreatitis
  - Helps in establishing the presence and extent of pancreatic necrosis (gas present) and local complications and to predict the severity of the disease
  - Also helps in assessing severity—by the CT-severity index
- MRI
  - MRCP—higher sensitivity for diagnosis of early acute pancreatitis
  - Better visualisation of pancreatic and bile ducts

Diagnosis

Severity determination

Modified Marshall's score

- Mild acute pancreatitis—absence of organ failure and local or systemic complications
- Moderately severe acute pancreatitis—transient organ failure (resolves within 48 hours) and/or local or systemic complications without persistent organ failure
- Severe acute pancreatitis—persistent organ failure (>48 hours) that may involve one or multiple organs

BISAP score

- B: BUN >25 mg/dL
- I: Impaired mental status
- S: SIRS

- A: Age >60 years
- P: Pleural effusion
- Presence of 3+—substantially increased risk for in-hospital mortality

MANAGEMENT

- 85–90% self limited,
- Subside spontaneously within 3–7 days of supportive treatment
  Nil per oral—to rest the pancreas
- Aggressive fluid resuscitation for hypotension:
  IV fluids – NS/RL at 15–20 mL/kg bolus (1000 ml to 1500 mL)
  – followed by 3 ml/kg/hr (around 200 ml/hr)
  – to maintain urine output at more than 0.5 ml/kg/hr
- For other patients 3–5 ml/kg/hr maintenance
  - Assess vitals, SpO_2, fluid status every few hours once—to decide on rate of fluid resuscitation
  - Monitor hematocrit and urea every 8 – 12 hours if increasing—repeat fluid bolus challenge
- IV analgesics—IV paracetamol (1 g IV q8 h), opioids (tramadol 50 mg q12 h – q8 h), NSAIDs (Lornoxicam 8 mg q12 h)
- Nutrition: Low-fat solid diet, soon after the pain has resolved in mild cases; in severe cases—enteral nutrition (gastric/nasojejunal) > TPN; maintains gut barrier integrity, limits bacterial translocation, less expensive, lesser complications
- No role for antibiotics (irrespective of fever and leukocytosis), unless there is a proof of infection

Specific Treatment

- Gallstone pancreatitis—ERCP within 24–48 hours of admission;
- Cholecystectomy after acute event resolves
- Hypertriglyceridemia—insulin infusion, heparin, plasmapheresis
- Treat the precipitating cause
- NSAIDs and pancreatic duct stenting-decreases incidence of post-ERCP pancreatitis

Complications

Local

- Acute peripancreatic fluid collection
- Necrosis—sterile/infected
- Pseudocyst formation
- Peripancreatic vascular complications—splenic vein thrombosis, pseudoaneurysm
- Pleural effusion
- Pancreatic ascitis

Systemic

- ARDS
- Pleural effusion
- Renal failure
- Cardiovascular collapse and hypotension.

Chapter

33

Hepatic Encephalopathy (HE)

Alteration in the mental status and cognitive function occurring in the presence of liver failure and/or porto-systemic shunting.

Can be secondary to acute liver failure, or more often due to chronic liver disease (cirrhosis)

Precipitating Factors

- Upper GI bleed
- Infections (especially spontaneous bacterial peritonitis and UTI)
- Hypokalemia and alkalosis (to look for diuretic use). It favours NH_3 production which crosses the blood–brain barrier and increases encephalopathy.
- Increased dietary proteins
- Constipation
- Sedatives

Signs and Symptoms

- Cirrhosis/hepatitis: Jaundice/ascites/splenomegaly
- Altered mental status: Either aggression or drowsiness
- Asterixis—flapping tremors is an important sign. Maybe absent as the patient becomes more drowsy.

West Haven Grading

Grade-1: Altered behavior, mild confusion, altered sleep-wake cycle
Grade-2: Moderate confusion, asterixis, lethargy, constructional apraxia
Grade-3: Marked confusion, asterixis stuporous
Grade-4: Deep coma

Investigations

- LFT
- RFT/sodium and potassium/HCO_3.
- CBP—to assess Hb drop for UGI bleed, TC for infection and platelet count
- Serum ammonia—may be elevated, but does not correlate to severity of encephalopathy. Normal levels do not rule out HE
- Ascitic tap—to rule out spontaneous bacterial peritonitis
- Blood culture, urine culture, CXR to judge source of infection

- EEG—bilaterally synchronous decrease in the wave frequency and increase in wave amplitude with loss of normal alpha-rhythm.

Treatment

- Correct precipitating factors:
  - Pass Ryle's tube and remove blood from upper GI if there is bleeding. This will go down to colon and act as substrate for bacteria. Control GI bleed (discussed in GI bleed chapter).
  - Start appropriate antibiotics after drawing blood cultures/ascitic fluid cultures/ urine cultures.
  - Correct K^+ levels as hypokalemia increases HE. Hydrate to avoid metabolic alkalosis.
  - Withdraw sedatives
  - Avoid constipation
- If agitated—antipsychotics to be administered with caution (preferred haloperidol, minimum dose starting from 1.25 to 5 mg /day)
- Proper dietary support (energy 40 kcal/kg/d and protein 1.2 g/kg/d); avoid protein restriction as it may promote muscle wasting and increase ammonia production.
- Animal protein should be avoided and switched to plant protein.
- Advice small meals with protein with a late night carbohydrate snack
- Lower ammonia level
  - Lactulose or lactitol 30 ml tid—titrate to pass 2 to 3 soft stools per day—acts by lowering colonic pH and reducing ammonia absorption, modifies colonic flora, cathartic effect to fasten GI transit time and to increase faecal nitrogen excretion. Can use up to 30 ml 2nd to 4th hourly
  - If this does not work, give lactulose enema, as alternative
  - Rifaximin (400 mg tid or 550 mg bd): Kills gut bacteria in colon which produce ammonia
  - Alternatives to rifaximin—metronidazole 400 mg tid, or amoxicillin 500 mg tid
  - L-ornithine L-aspartate(IV/oral)—enhances metabolism of ammonia to glutamine.
- Chronic hepatic encephalopathy:

  Some patients may require continuation of rifaximin and lactulose for longer periods if they have chronic hepatic encephalopathy.

Chapter

34

Spontaneous Bacterial Peritonitis (SBP)

- Ascitic fluid infection without an intra-abdominal surgical source.
- Most common organism is *E. coli*.
- Klebsiella, Streptococcus, Staphylococcus also known.

Evidence of SBP

1. **Monobacterial ascitic fluid shows ≥250 neutrophils with culture growing an organism.**
2. **Culture negative neutrophilic**—culture sterile but ascitic fluid differential count shows ≥250 polymorphs.
3. **Monobacterial non-neutrophilic**—culture grows an organism but ascitic fluid count does not show ≥250 neutrophils
4. **Polymicrobial**—when culture grows more than one organism.

Pathophysiology

Translocation of gut microorganisms.

Cirrhosis of liver predisposes to:

- Bacterial overgrowth in the small intestine
- Increased permeability of the intestinal walls

Risk factors for SBP in cirrhosis.

- Ascitic fluid total protein concentration < 1 g/dL
- Prior episode of SBP
- Variceal hemorrhage is an important factor
- Serum total bilirubin concentration above 2.5 mg/dL, in cirrhotic patients

Clinical Features

Most common symptoms are:

- Fever
- Pain abdomen—diffuse, continuous, associated with tenderness.
- Altered mental status—due to infection or hepatic encephalopathy
- Diarrhea

More severe symptoms include—hypotension and paralytic ileus.

Diagnosis of SBP

- CBP: Increased total count, raised neutrophil count, peripheral smear—may show toxic granules
- LFT-for cirrhosis, especially serum albumin to calculate serum ascites albumin fluid gradient (SAAG)
- RFT/serum electrolytes—hepatorenal syndrome is common in SBP
- Blood culture—for sepsis

Ascitic Fluid Analysis

- Total count > 250 polymorphoneutrophils (PMN)
- Culture—10 ml of fluid is sent for culture
- Serum ascites albumin gradient (SAAG): High SAAG is suggestive of portal hypertension and is more likely associated with SBP.
- Protein—lower ascitic fluid protein is associated with SBP.
- LDH—with increased neutrophils, cell lysis increases and ascites fluid LDH increases.

Treatment

- Empirical antibiotics after paracentesis and drawing cultures (no need to wait for results).
- Cefotaxime 2 g IV 8th hourly is preferred. Ceftriaxone 2 g IV od is also used.
- Switch to appropriate antibiotics after culture is available.
- In case fluid shows <250 neutrophils, but strong suspicion of SBP antibiotics are started in symptomatic individuals and repeat tap is done after 48 hours in asymptomatic individuals.
- Duration of antibiotics is 5–7 days.
- In case fever persists after 7 days, repeat ascitic fluid analysis is done to look for polymorphs.
- Stop beta blockers—may cause more HRS.
- If hepatorenal syndrome develops, treat appropriately.
- Ciprofloxacin 400 mg IV bd can be used in case cephalosporins cannot be used but is avoided if the individual was already on SBP prophylaxis with quniolones.

Prophylaxis

General measures for future management:

- Diuretics—to make the ascitic fluid more concentrated and improving opsonin activity in it.
- Restricting proton pump inhibitors.
- Early recognition and aggressive treatment of infections.

Antibiotic Prophylaxis

Required in:

- Patients with cirrhosis and UGI bleed.
- Patients who have had previous episodes of SBP.
- Ascitic fluid albumin <1.5 g with live failure (child pugh score >9) or renal failure.

Dose (till ascites resolves)

- Norflox 400 mg od
- Ciprofloxacin 500 mg od
- Co-trimoxazole DS 1 tablet od—for 5 days in a week

Chapter

35

Hepatorenal Syndrome (HRS)

Hepatorenal syndrome is defined as development of renal failure in patients with advanced liver failure (acute or chronic) ***in the absence of any identifiable causes of renal pathology***.

Diagnosis of exclusion, when all other causes of renal failure, functional or organic, have been excluded.

Types

- Type 1 HRS—two fold increase in serum creatinine to >2.5 mg/dL or 50 percent reduction in creatinine clearance during a period of <2 weeks
- Type 2 HRS—is defined as renal impairment that is less severe than with type 1 disease and occurs over >2 weeks.

Pathogenesis

Cirrhosis of liver—causes increased nitric oxide levels in the splanchnic system (decreased clearance and bacterial translocation)

- Causes splanchnic vasodilation. This leads to a hyperdynamic state
- Sympathetic system and RAS activation causes renal vasoconstriction

  The systemic hypotension and renal vasoconstriction cause decrease in GFR.

Precipitating Factors

- Diuretic therapy
- Spontaneous bacterial peritonitis
- Large volume paracentesis
- Gastrointestinal bleeding
- Superimposed alcoholic hepatitis
- Infections causing sepsis

Clinical Features

I. Type 1 (more serious):

- Rapid and progressive deterioration/oliguria and rising creatinine
- Patient is ill with severe cirrhosis of liver, jaundice and hyponatremia
- Hepatic encephalopathy present
- Hypovolemic: Tachycardia, hypotension and precordial systolic murmur
- Massive ascites +/– pedal edema

II. Type 2 (less serious)

- Relatively stable serum creatinine that gradually increases over months
- Usually stable Child-Pugh-B with preserved liver function
- Mild jaundice, some degree of coagulopathy
- No hepatic encephalopathy
- Urine output is maintained for months

The International ascites club diagnostic criteria for HRS is:

- Cirrhosis with ascites
- Serum creatinine >1.5 mg/dL or rise in creatinine >0.3mg/dL within 48 hours or 1.5 times the baseline value
- No improvement of serum creatinine (decrease to a level of 1.5 mg/dL) after at least 2 days of diuretic withdrawal and volume expansion with albumin (20% 1gm/kg/day)
- Absence of shock
- No current or recent treatment with nephrotoxic drugs
- Absence of parenchymal kidney disease as indicated by proteinuria <500 mg/day, and/or normal renal ultrasonography (thus ruling out underlying renal disease)

INVESTIGATIONS

- A progressive **rise in serum creatinine** with or without oliguria
  But normal renal functioning as shown by:
  - A normal urine sediment
  - No or minimal proteinuria (<500 mg per day)
  - Urine sodium <10 mEq/L (shows normal concentrating capacity of kidney)
- LFT—consistent with cirrhosis of liver (low albumin, high globulin)
- USG abdomen—for cirrhosis, ascites and to rule out chronic kidney disease
- CBP and appropriate cultures to rule out infection

Management

- Treatment of cause is important for recovery of liver function.
- Treat with antivirals for hepatitis, withdrawal from alcohol for alcoholic liver disease.

Meanwhile, the following are done:

- Workup to rule out other causes of renal disease
- Fluid challenge to treat subclinical hypovolemia
- Precipitants should be identified and corrected
- Sepsis workup and cultures to be sent

To improve systemic hemodynamics:

- **For critically ill with hypotension (noradrenaline plus albumin)**
  - Noradrenaline: Dose: 0.1 to 3 μg/kg/min
  - Dilution: Taken as 8 mg (1 ml = 1 mg). 8 ml in 42 ml normal saline. It can be started at 2 ml/hr (0.1 μg/kg/min) and can increased to 22 ml/hr (1 μg/kg/min)
  - Vasopressin infusion: Dose—0.03 units/minute

    - 40 units/ml. Dilute 1 ml in 39 ml normal saline. It can be started at 1.2 ml/hr (0.02 units/minute) and increased to 2.4 ml/hr (0.04 units/minute).
  - **PLUS:** Albumin—1g/kg/d (maximum 100 g/d) for 2 days
- Duration of treatment is 2 weeks
- **Not critically ill (terlipressin plus albumin)**
  Terlipressin—1–2 mg q4 h to q6 h as IV bolus plus
  Albumin—1g/kg/d (max 100 g/d) for 2 days, followed by 25–50 g/d, till terlipressin is discontinued
- Alternate—midodrine/octreotide with albumin
  Midodrine—oral 7.5 mg q8 h – uptitrated to maximum 15 mg q8 h
  Octreotide—continuous IV infusion (50 μg/hr) or S/C 100–200 μg q8 h

Other treatment options

- Dialysis may be needed in the waiting period for liver transplant
- TIPS—transjugular intrahepatic porto-systemic shunt
- Extracorporeal albumin dialysis
- Liver transplantation

Prognosis

Depends on liver function

Generally poor prognosis, unless there is a reversible cause like diuretic therapy.

Section

5

Renal Injury, Acid–Base Disorders and Electrolytes Imbalance

Chapter

36

Acute Kidney Injury

Definition

Abrupt decline in GFR which leads to decreased elimination of nitrogenous waste from the kidney.

Acute kidney injury (AKI) is defined as any of the following:

- Increase in serum creatinine by >0.3 mg/dl within 48 hours.
- Increase in serum creatinine to >1.5 times baseline, occurred within the prior 7 days.
- Urine volume < 0.5 mL/kg/h for 6 hours.

Stages of AKI

1. KDIGO (Kidney Disease: Improving Global Outcomes) criteria:

	Serum creatinine	**Urine output**
Stage 1	1.5 to 1.9 times baseline/rise of 0.3 mg/dL	<0.5 mL/kg/hour in 6–12 hours
Stage 2	2–2.9 times baseline	<0.5 mL/kg/hour for >12 hours
Stage 3	3 times baseline or increase in serum creatinine >4 mg/dL, or initiation of renal replacement therapy	<0.3 mL/kg/hour >24 hours or anuria >12 hours

Other staging include:

2. RIFLE (risk, injury, failure, loss, end stage renal disease) criteria
3. AKIN (acute kidney injury network) criteria

Causes of AKI

A. Prerenal causes

- Hypovolemia
- Cardiac failure
- Hepatorenal syndrome

B. Renal causes

1. Vascular
   - Malignant HTN
   - Renal artery stenosis
   - Large or medium vessel vasculitis

2. Glomerular disease
   - Lupus nephritis/postinfectious glomerulonephritis
3. Acute tubular necrosis
   - Ischemia
   - Nephrotoxins
   - Rhabdomyolysis
4. Acute interstitial nephritis
   - Drugs

C. Postrenal causes

- BPH
- Renal calculi

Clinical Examination

- Edema +
- BP: Low in pre renal causes and septic shock/raised in established renal failure
- RR: Increased in acidotic breathing, pulmonary edema
- Raised JVP
- Bilateral basal crepitations—for pulmonary edema
- Altered sensorium and asterixis—uremic encephalopathy
- Palpable bladder—in urethral obstruction in benign prostatic hypertrophy

Investigations

CBP—to rule out sepsis
Peripheral smear schistocytes—TTP, HUS
Blood/urine cultures—for sepsis

Urine

- Normal—in prerenal and postrenal AKI
- Casts and sediments—protein+, RBCs + in renal causes of AKI
- Urine sodium <20 mmol/L in prerenal
  >40 mmol/L in renal
  Fractional excretion of Na <1% in prerenal; >1% in ATN

Biochemistry

- Urea/creatinine increased.
- UR/CR ratio increased in prerenal AKI
- Sodium/potassium—may be raised
- Serum bicarbonate—low, metabolic acidosis
- Calcium low/phosphorus maybe high-mild
- Uric acid—high
- CK—high in rhabdomyolysis
- ABG—for pH being low-metabolic acidosis, hypoxia—due to pulmonary edema

Chest X-ray—for pulmonary edema
ECG—for hyperkalemia

Ultrasound for kidneys

- Normal size in pre renal and renal causes
- Shrunken in AKI on CKD
- May show obstructive uropathy in postrenal—BPH, hydronephrosis, etc.

Management

Principles of Therapy

1. Correct reversible causes which are treatable
2. Avoid potential insults
3. Metabolic support till kidneys recover
4. Management of complications

1. Correct reversible causes

- Treat sepsis with appropriate antibiotics
- Relieving obstruction—stenting for ureteric obstruction/operate BPH, etc.
- Treating hypovolemia-with fluids

If hypovolemic

- 1.5 – 3L of NS can be given.
- In case of fluid responders (urine output of 0.5 mL/kg/hr), fluids are continued at 75 mL/hour.
- In case of non-responders, ATN should be thought of and progressive volume expansion avoided.
- If fluid status is difficult to assess, 1 L of crystalloid IV fluid is given, and the patient is assessed for response.

Cardiac failure—treat with diuretics and inotropes.

2. Avoid potential insults

- Avoid nephrotoxic drugs—ACE inhibitors, ARB, NSAIDS, aminoglycosides
- Modification of doses of drugs as per GFR
- Avoiding iodinated contrast
- Avoiding hypotension
- The doses of renally excreted drugs has to be modified after calculating the GFR
- The formulae used are as follows:
  - Cockcroft-Gault equation
  - $\text{CrCl, mL/min} = \dfrac{(140 - \text{age}) \times (\text{weight in kg})}{(72 \times \text{Cr})} \times (0.85 \text{ if female})$
  - Other formulae used: CKD-EPI, MDRD equation

3. General supportive measures

Fluid management

- Strict intake output chart
- Daily weight monitoring
- Intake = output on previous day + 500 mL

If hypervolemic

- Initially 80 mg of frusemide is given IV
- In case the patient is already receiving diuretics at home, double the dose is given.
- 200 mL of urine over the next 2 hours after IV diuretics is considered a good response.
- Lack of response predicts the need for dialysis
- In case of an augmented response after 2 hours, the diuretic dose can be doubled and repeated.

Diet:

- Restrict protein intake: 0.5 g/kg of high biological value
- Restrict salt intake to <5 g/day, if fluid overloaded
- Avoid high potassium diet

Other measures:

- Hypotension—inotropic support
- Uremic gastritis—Inj pantoprazole 40 mg IV od
- Catheterise unconscious patient/patient with urethral obstruction
- Care of unconscious patient

4. Management of complications (refer to chapters on these topics for details)

- Pulmonary edema: If BP > 120/80 mm of Hg, 80–200 mg IV frusemide . If the patient is hypoxic, give oxygen supplementation. If needed, intubation and ventilation
- Hyperkalemia—antihyperkalemic measures
- IV bicarbonate correction—refer to chapter on metabolic acidosis
- Hypertension—all antihypertensive drugs can be used, except ACE -I, and ARBs
- Hypocalcemia and hyperphosphatemia—refer to relevant chapters.

Urgent hemodialysis

- Refractory pulmonary edema with oliguria
- Refractory hyperkalemia >6 mEq/dL after correction
- Metabolic acidosis (pH<7.1)—unless acidosis can be rapidly corrected by correction of underlying etiology.
- Altered sensorium due to uremia.
- Acute poisoning
- Oliguria

Note

- Hemodialysis is risky when blood pressure is not maintained, and may fall during dialysis.
- Patients may need inotropic support to go through the procedure.
- The absolute value of creatinine is not an indication for dialysis.

If the BP is low, and patient needs dialysis, the either of following procedures can be adopted:

- SLED—sustained low efficiency dialysis
  - Removes fluid over 6–8 hours.
  - Slower removal, hence less hemodynamic instability

- CRRT—continuous renal replacement therapy
  - Removes fluids over 24 hours,very slowly.
  - Useful when a patient is very fluid overloaded, needs more fluid removal, but this cannot be done fast, as the patient has hypotension and is on inotropes.
  - Also done when patient needs to be given fluids, like on TPN, or needs blood component replacement for another indication.
  - Is better than SLED on the fluid status, but is more expensive and equipment may not be available.

Monitoring

- Body weight daily
- Intake/output daily
- Urea/creatinine, Na/K/HCO_3 daily

Recovery

- Increase in urine output may be first sign of recovery
- Urea/creatinine may fall after 1–2 days
- Dialysis may need to be continued based on clinical and biochemical parameters till recovery.

Management during Diuretic Phase

Patient may have high output, and also lose electrolytes.

Fluid Management

- Fluid may be increased based on monitored output
- Oral or IV fluids may be needed to avoid dehydration, and this will again cause rise in creatinine.

Supplementation of Na and K may be advised if levels fall.

Chapter

37 Interpretation of Arterial Blood Gas (ABG) for Acid–Base Disorders

Arterial blood gas analysis is done by drawing an arterial blood sample from the radial artery. It gives information on the pH, PaO_2 (arterial oxygen content), $PaCO_2$ (carbon dioxide content), and HCO_3 (bicarbonate levels) in the arterial blood. It is very useful in detecting acid–base disorders, and respiratory failure.

NORMAL VALUES

- pH: 7.35–7.45
- PaO_2: 85–100 mm Hg
- $PaCO_2$: 35–45 mmHg
- HCO_3: 21–27 mEq/L
  - Age correction for PaO_2 is 100 (1/3 × patient's age). Example: In a 60 year old patient, expected PaO_2 is 100 (1/3 × 60) = 80 mm of Hg.
  - The last two digits of pH and the $PaCO_2$ are the same (7.35 to 7.45 and 35–45 mm of Hg).

Differences between ABG and VBG

- The arterial and venous values are **not significantly different** for practical purposes except in the cases of PO_2 and $PaCO_2$.
- Peripheral venous pH is only **0.02 to 0.04 lower** than the arterial pH.
- Peripheral venous HCO_3 concentration is approximately 1 to 2 mEq/L higher than the arterial HCO_3.
- Venous PO_2 is 36.9 mmHg lower than arterial, and hence cannot be trusted.

APPROACH TO DIAGNOSIS OF ACID–BASE DISORDERS

1. Diagnose the Primary Disorder

Look at pH

Acidosis: pH <7.35

To decide whether the acidosis is respiratory or metabolic, look at $PaCO_2$.

- If $PaCO_2$ is high-respiratory acidosis
- HCO_3 is low-metabolic acidosis

Alkalosis: pH >7.45

- If $PaCO_2$ is low-respiratory alkalosis
- If HCO_3 is high-metabolic alkalosis

pH	$PaCO_2$	Primary disorder	Compensation
⇩	⇩	Metabolic acidosis (↓ HCO_3)	↓ $PaCO_2$
⇧	⇧	Metabolic alkalosis (↑ HCO_3)	↑ $PaCO_2$
⇩	⇧	Respiratory acidosis (↑ $PaCO_2$)	↑ HCO_3
⇧	⇩	Respiratory alkalosis (↓ $PaCO_2$)	↓ HCO_3

a. If pH and $PaCO_2$ move in the same direction the primary disorder is metabolic.

b. If pH and $PaCO_2$ move in the opposite direction the primary disorder is respiratory. Compensatory response is dependent on the type of primary disorder.

2 Calculating Compensation

An underlying acid–base disorder may have a normal pH if it is compensated. **The changes in $PaCO_2$ and HCO_3 in opposite directions indicate a mixed acid–base disorder.**

Primary disorder	Compensation
Metabolic acidosis	Expected $PaCO_2 = (1.5 \times HCO_3) + 8 +/- 2$ (or) **Winter's formula, or** $PaCO_2 = HCO_3 + 15$ (works for $PaCO_2$ between 10 and 40) or 1.2 mmHg decrease in $PaCO_2$ for every 1 mmol/L decrease in HCO_3.
Metabolic alkalosis	0.7 mmHg increase in $PaCO_2$ for every 1 mmol/L increase in HCO_3.
Respiratory acidosis	
Acute compensation	$HCO_3 = 24 + (\text{actual } PaCO_2 - 40) \div 10$ For every 10 mmHg rise in $PaCO_2$, HCO_3 increases by **1 mmol/L**
Chronic compensation	$HCO_3 = 24 + 4 (\text{actual } PaCO_2 - 40) \div 10$ For every 10 mmHg rise in $PaCO_2$, HCO_3 increases by **4 mmol/L**
Respiratory alkalosis	
Acute compensation	$HCO_3 = 24 + 2 (\text{Actual } PaCO_2 - 40) \div 10$ For every 10 mmHg fall in $PaCO_2$, HCO_3 decreases by **2 mmol/L**
Chronic compensation	$HCO_3 = 24 + 4 (\text{actual } PaCO_2 - 40) \div 10$ For every 10 mmHg fall in $PaCO_2$, HCO_3 decreases by **4 mmol/L**

3. Calculate Anion Gap

This is a vital step in interpreting an ABG and should never be missed as there are mixed acid–base disorders which may have normal pH and HCO_3 and can only be diagnosed by looking at the anion gap.

Anion gap = Na-(Cl + HCO_3)

Normal range = 8–10 mmol/L

Changes in Anion Gap

Causes for low anion gap:
1. Addition of abnormal cations (lithium intoxication, plasma cell dyscrasia)
2. Reduced albumin (nephrotic syndrome, chronic liver disease, malabsorption)
3. Hyperviscosity and hyperlipidemia (causes underestimation of Na and Cl)

Correction for Hypoalbuminemia

For every 1gm/dL decrease in serum albumin, **2.5 mmol/L** should be added to the anion gap.

Based on the anion gap, metabolic acidosis is classified to be high anion gap acidosis and normal anion gap acidosis.

Important

1. While drawing ABG, avoid air bubbles in the syringe.
2. All ABG must be interpreted in the context of clinical background.
3. Additional information about RBS, electrolytes, albumin, etc. will be needed to avoid errors in interpretation.
4. Treatment of cause may correct many acid–base disorders, which may not require treatment on their own merit.

APPROACH TO INTERPRETATION OF HYPOXIA AND HYPERCARBIA

Check PaO_2: Low PaO_2 indicates respiratory failure

Type 1 respiratory failure

- PaO_2 is low
- $PaCO_2$ is normal or low

Type 2 respiratory failure

- PaO_2 is low
- $PaCO_2$ is high

Causes of acute type 1 respiratory failure

- Pneumonia
- Bronchial asthma
- ARDS
- Pulmonary edema
- Pulmonary embolism

Causes of chronic type 1 respiratory failure

- Interstitial lung disease
- Pure emphysema

Causes of acute type 2 respiratory failure

Upper airway obstruction

- Laryngeal edema/foreign body/strangulation

Causes of acute hypoventilation

- Respiratory center depression—sedatives and poisons/strokes/meningoencephalitis
- Neuromuscular paralysis—GBS/OP poisoning/myasthenia/snake bite
- COPD—acute exacerbations
- late ARDS/severe asthma

Causes of chronic type 2 respiratory failure

- COPD
- Chest wall deformities

Note

All type 1 respiratory failures can become type 2, with rise in CO_2, in late stages.

Chapter

38

Acidosis

Acidosis is classified into metabolic acidosis if HCO_3 is low, and respiratory acidosis if pCO_2 is high.

METABOLIC ACIDOSIS

Metabolic acidosis is diagnosed if pH is <7.36 and HCO_3 < 21 mEq/dL.
It is classified on the basis of anion gap into
- Normal anion gap metabolic acidosis (NAGMA)
- High anion gap metabolic acidosis (HAGMA).

Causes of Normal Anion Gap Metabolic Acidosis (NAGMA)

1. Increased GI bicarbonate loss

A. Diarrhea

B. External pancreatic or small bowel drainage

C. Ureterosigmoidostomy, jejunal loop, ileal loop

D. *Drugs*—magnesium sulfate, cholestyramine, calcium chloride

2. Renal tubular acidosis (RTA)

With hypokalemia:

a. Proximal RTA(type 2)

b. Distal RTA (type 1)

With hyperkalemia:

a. Type 4 RTA

b. Chronic kidney disease

3. Drug induced

a. Potassium sparing diuretics (amiloride, triamterene, spironolactone, eplerenone)

b. Trimethoprim

c. ACE inhibitors and ARBs

d. NSAIDs

e. Calcineurin inhibitors

4. Others

A. Expansion acidosis (rapid saline administration)

B. Loss of potential HCO_3 (excretion of ketones in ketoacidosis)

Causes of high anion gap metabolic acidosis (HAGMA)

Mnemonic: **CAT MUDPILES**

C: Cyanide or carbon monoxide

A: Acetaminophen, aspirin, alcoholic ketoacidosis

T: Toluene

M: Methanol

U: Uremia

D: Diabetic ketoacidosis

P: Propylene glycol

I: Isoniazid, iron

L: Lactic acidosis

E: Ethylene glycol

S: Salicylates

DELTA GAP RATIO

In the presence of a high AG acidosis, calculate the delta-gap to diagnose an additional mixed disorder.

This is calculated by the ratio between the increase in anion gap and the decrease in HCO_3.

$$\text{Delta gap ratio} = \frac{\text{Anion gap} - 12}{24\text{-}HCO_3 \text{ level}}$$

If <0.4 pure $NAGMA_2$
If 0.4 – 0.8 mixed NAGMA + HAGMA
If 0.8 – 2.0 pure HAGMA
If >2.0 mixed HAGMA + metabolic alkalosis

Clinical features of metabolic acidosis

- Unusual weakness, fatigue
- acidotic breathing—Kussmaul's breathing—deep sighing respiration in the context of normal oxygen saturation
- Features of underlying cause such as DKA, uremia/sepsis
- Hypotension
- Confusion/coma

MANAGEMENT

The treatment of metabolic acidosis primarily involves the correction of the underlying cause. The need for alkali therapy is as follows:

Firstly, it is important to recognize if the acidosis is acute or chronic.

Alkali therapy is indicated in acute acidemia-

→ Severe acute acidemia (pH <7.1)

→ Acute acidemia (7.1–7.2) with acute kidney injury (oliguria or rise in creatinine)

Calculation of deficit:

- Alkali deficit = 0.5 × body weight × (desired HCO_3 – actual HCO_3)
- Half of the deficit to be given over 1 hour, and the rest over 24 hours.

Alkali therapy

- $NaHCO_3$ is available as 50 mL vial of 8.4% (50 mEq/50 mL) or 7.5% (44.6 mEq/50 mL) and each vial can raise the serum HCO_3 by 1.3 to 1.5 mEq/L
- As there is a risk of raising sodium levels, the alkali therapy if more than two vials are to be administered it is usually given as infusion with 5% dextrose.
- Initial administration of 50 mEq of $NaHCO_3$ diluted in 300 mL can be given over 30 mins during the initial 1–2 hours of therapy and the target pH being ~7.2.
- Conversely 3 vials of $NaHCO_3$ can be diluted in 1 L of 5% dextrose and administered over 3 hours.

LACTIC ACIDOSIS

Type A (poor tissue perfusion)

1. Cardiogenic, septic, hypovolemic shock
2. Severe anemia
3. Mitochondrial enzyme defects and inhibitors (cyanide, carbon monoxide)

Type B

1. Hepatic failure
2. Malignancy
3. Drugs:
   - Metformin
   - Ethylene glycol, methanol, propylene glycol, ethanol
   - Propofol
   - Stavudine, didanosine

Management

1. Treat cause
2. Tissue perfusion should be restored adequately.
3. Adequate ventilation: If required intubation may be done to achieve this.
4. Goal in non-intubated patients with severe acidemia: An appropriate ventilatory response should reduce the partial pressure of carbon dioxide (PCO_2) to at least 15 mmHg and often to 10 to 12 mmHg.
5. Indication for bicarbonate: Ventilation adequate, but severe lactic acidosis (pH less than 7.1).

Dose

- IV sodium bicarbonate bolus of 1 to 2 mEq/kg body weight.
- Measure serum electrolytes and blood pH 30 to 60 minutes later, and the dose of sodium bicarbonate can be repeated if severe lactic acidosis (pH less than 7.1) persists.
- Watch for fall in calcium and potassium with bicarbonate administration.

RESPIRATORY ACIDOSIS

ETIOLOGY

1. Pulmonary Disorders (Parenchymal/Airway/Gas Exchange Abnormalities)

1. Chronic obstructive pulmonary disease
2. Severe asthma
3. Upper respiratory obstruction
   A. Severe laryngeal or tracheal—stenosis/edema/ tumors
   B. Obstructive sleep apnea

2. Decreased Central Respiratory Drive

1. Sedative overdose (benzodiazepines, tricyclic antidepressants, narcotics)
2. CNS disorders—encephalopathy due to any cause, brainstem stroke
3. Obstructive sleep apnea.

3. Decreased Respiratory Function (Neuromuscular or Thoracic Abnormalities)

Neuromuscular

1. Guillain-Barré syndrome
2. Cervical spine injury/disease
3. Myasthenia gravis
4. Tick paralysis
5. Periodic paralysis

Thoracic abnormalities

1. Kyphoscoliosis
2. Flail chest
3. Ankylosing spondylitis
4. Obesity hypoventilation syndrome (OHS)

Clinical Features

The clinical features vary according to the severity and duration of the respiratory acidosis, the underlying disease, and whether there is accompanying severe hypoxemia.

The following are the features of high $PaCO_2$:

1. Drowsiness, tiredness
2. Dyspnea
3. Headache
4. Coma

Signs of CO_2 narcosis

1. Flushed skin/warm peripheries
2. Bounding pulse
3. **Asterixis** (flapping tremors)
4. Papilledema

Lesser degrees of dysfunction in chronic hypercapnia include

1. Daytime somnolence
2. Impairment of coordination
3. Motor disturbances such as tremor, myoclonic jerks, and asterixis

MANAGEMENT

Arterial blood gas analysis

- A low pH (<7.35)
- High pCO_2 (>45 mm Hg)
- Further evaluation should be done to differentiate between acute and chronic respiratory acidosis which is based on the underlying history.
- **Acute respiratory acidosis**
  - pH is low
  - pCO_2 is raised
  - $[HCO_3^-]$ which increases 1 mmol/L for every 10 mmHg increase in $PaCO_2$.
- **Chronic respiratory acidosis (2–3 days)**
  - pH may be low normal/normal (7.33–7.35) due to renal compensation increasing HCO_3
  - pCO_2 is raised
  - $[HCO_3^-]$ increased by 4 mmol/L for every 10 mmHg increase in $PaCO_2$.

Assess airway and breathing

1. Administer oxygen if patient has low saturation (<90%)

   Caution: In patients of COPD with type 2 respiratory failure target saturation between 90–93%. Do not aim for higher O_2 targets.

   Higher saturation can cause hypercapnia due to reduced respiratory drive (COPD patients depend on hypoxia for the respiratory drive)
2. Noninvasive ventilation for mild-moderate respiratory failure, i.e, for example, in patients of COPD with preserved consciousness (refer to chapter on COPD on details of ventilation)
3. Severe respiratory distress and/or marked hemodynamic instability : Intubate.
4. Upper airway obstruction: Emergency tracheostomy
5. Simultaneously the definitive treatment such as bronchodilators and antibiotics should be initiated to treat the underlying etiology.

Chapter

39

Alkalosis

Metabolic Alkalosis

- Arterial pH >7.45, or
- Serum bicarbonate >30 mmol/L.

Important to note:

- Any bicarbonate level above 35 mmol/L is not a simple compensation for respiratory acidosis. True alkalosis exists above this level.
- Hypokalemia causes metabolic alkalosis, by intracellular H^+ shift, and renal H^+ loss.

Causes

- Gastrointestinal H^+ loss
  - Vomiting
  - Nasogastric suction
  - Villous adenomas
  - High-volume ileostomy losses
- Renal H^+ loss
  - Diuretics
  - Steroids
  - Bartter syndrome and Gitelman syndrome
  - Mineralocorticoid excess
  - Primary hyperaldosteronism
  - Liddle syndrome
  - Posthypercapnia
- Other causes
  - Contraction alkalosis: Any volume depleted state
  - Alkali intake or administration, milk-alkali syndrome
  - Hypokalemia
  - Massive blood transfusion or FFP transfusion (due to citrate)

Clinical Features

- Usually asymptomatic
- Symptoms due to—
  - Hypokalemia: Paresthesia, cramping, fatigue and arrhythmia

- Bicarbonate >45 mmol/L, causes hypoventilation, hypoxemia, especially in COPD patients
- Bicarbonate >50 mmol/L: Seizures, altered mental status, and coma.

Investigations

- ABG—will show
  - pH to be more than 7.45
  - HCO_3 of more than 30 mmol/L
- $PaCO_2$ compensation:
  - PCO_2 will increase by 0.7 mmHg for each 1 mmol/L rise of HCO_3
  - Serum electrolytes—serum potassium is low
- Urine chloride levels:
  - If less than 10 mmol/L—suggestive of chloride responsive disorders such as vomiting, etc.
  - If more than 30 mmol/L other causes such as mineralocorticoid excess should be thought of.

Treatment

- Treat the underlying causes—vomiting, diuretic dose should be reduced or stopped.
- In chloride depletion and contraction alkalosis: Start on IV normal saline.
- In edematous states (CCF) give K^+ correction and K^+ sparing diuretics.
  - Spironolactone (start at 12.5 mg or 25 mg od, increased to a max of 50 mg)
  - Eplerenone (start at 25 mg and increase to 50 mg od) until K normalizes.
  - Acetazolamide 250 to 500 mg, od or bd, can be tried for additional diuresis
- For posthypercapnic alkalosis: Acetazolamide 250 mg od
- Hypokalemia: Should be corrected either orally or intravenously.
- Treatment of primary hyperaldosteronism: Use spironolactone and eplerenone.
- Rarely: HCL infusion

Respiratory Alkalosis

- pH > 7.45
- pCO_2< 35 mmHg due to hyperventilation.

Causes

- Hypoxemia or tissue hypoxia
  - Decreased inspired oxygen tension
  - Bacterial or viral pneumonia, aspiration pneumonia
  - Pulmonary embolism
  - Drowning
  - Pulmonary edema/CCF
- Central nervous system stimulation
  - Voluntary
  - Pain and anxiety syndrome

  - Fever
  - Raised ICT—subarachnoid hemorrhage and tumor
- Miscellaneous
  - Pregnancy
  - Mechanical hyperventilation
  - Salicylate overdose
  - Recovery from metabolic acidosis

Signs and Symptoms of Respiratory Alkalosis

- Central nervous system (in acute respiratory alkalosis)
  - Light-headedness
  - Confusion
  - Generalized seizures
- Cardiovascular system: Cardiac arrhythmias
- Neuromuscular system: Due to decrease in ionised calcium due to alkalosis
  - Numbness and paresthesia of the extremities
  - Circumoral numbness
  - Laryngeal spasm
  - Manifestations of tetany muscle cramps—carpopedal spasm, Trousseau's sign, and Chvostek's sign.

Investigations

- Arterial blood gas analysis
  - pH >7.45
  - Reduced $PaCO_2$
- HCO_3 compensation
  - Acute alkalosis: HCO_3 reduces by 2 mmol/L for every 10 mm drop in $PaCO_2$
  - Chronic alkalosis compensation: HCO_3 reduces by 4 mmol/L for every 10 mm drop in $PaCO_2$
  - Hypoxia: Low PaO_2 as a cause of hyperventilation
- Serum electrolytes: Reduced ionized calcium and serum potassium
- Investigations to evaluate the primary cause for hyperventilation(both respiratory and neurological)

Treatment

- Underlying cause should be identified and treated specifically
- Psychiatric causes such as anxiety and stress, can have voluntary hyperventilation and may benefit from reassurance, rebreathing masks and attention to the underlying psychological factors.

Chapter

40

Hyperkalemia

Normal serum potassium levels range from 3.5 to 5 mEq/L.

- Mild hyperkalemia—5 to 6 mEq/L
- Moderate hyperkalemia—6 to 7 mEq/L
- Severe hyperkalemia— >7 mEq/L

A total body K^+ excess of 100–200 mEq is required to produce 1 mEq/L increase in plasma K.

Causes of Hyperkalemia

Increased potassium release from cells	Reduced urinary potassium excretion
Pseudohyperkalemia—hemolyzed sample	Reduced aldosterone secretion
Metabolic acidosis	Reduced response to aldosterone
Insulin deficiency	Acute kidney injury
Hyperosmolality	Chronic kidney disease
Increased tissue catabolism—rhabdomyolysis hemolysis/crush injuries/tumor lysis	ACE inhibitors, potassium sparing diuretics type 4 RTA
Beta blockers	Addison's disease
Blood transfusions/K infusions with IV fluids	

Clinical Manifestations

- Maybe asymptomatic
- Fatigue
- Paresthesias
- Palpitations
- Severe muscle weakness or paralysis—can cause ascending paralysis
- Cardiac manifestations—arrhythmias, asystole and death.

Investigations

Biochemistry

- Random blood sugar
  - Urea/creatinine—for renal failure
  - Serum bicarbonate—for acidosis
  - ABG—if RTA is suspected

ECG changes: Note: May not always reflect serum K level

K > 5.5–6.5 mEq/L (repolarization abnormalities)

- Tented tall t waves—narrow base and sharp tips of tall T waves

K > 6.5–7mEq/L (atrial paralysis)

- P waves widens and flattens, PR segment lengthens, p waves eventually disappear-

K > 7–9 mEq/L (conduction blocks)

- Bradyarrhythmias
- Prolonged QRS complex, AV block

K >9 mEq/L

- Development of sine wave, wide complex, asystole, ventricular fibrillation, pulseless electrical activity.

Management

Patients with hyperkalemic emergency should be identified so that immediate lifesaving therapy can be initiated:

Antagonism of membrane actions • Calcium gluconate
Drive potassium into the cell • Insulin and glucose • Sodium bicarbonate • Beta 2 adrenergic agonists
Removal of potassium from the body • Loop or thiazide diuretics • Cation exchange resins • Dialysis

1. In mild hyperkalemia:
    - Stop all potassium containing foods: Fruits, nuts, lentils, spinach and tomatoes.
    - Stop all medications that can increase potassium, e.g. ACE inhibitors and beta blockers
    - Give potassium binding resin—sodium polystyrene sulfonate 15 to 30 g PO tid. It can also be given as retention enema.
    - Correct acidosis with 100 mL of 8.4% sodium bicarbonate over 15 minutes (weak effect)
2. In moderate and severe hyperkalemia (most act within 20–30 minutes)
    a. 50 mL of 50% glucose IV with 10 units of insulin IV. Watch for hypo- or hyperglycemia.
    b. Correct acidosis with 100 mL of 8.4% sodium bicarbonate over 15 minutes.
    c. IV 10% calcium gluconate 10 mL over 10 minutes if ECG changes are present. This needs other measures, as it does not reduce serum levels, but stabilises the heart.
    d. Inj frusemide 40 mg IV stat and 12th hourly if renal function is not severely impaired.
    e. Beta 2 agonist nebulisation—salbutamol approximetely 4 times the therapeutic dose—20 mg– over 10 minutes—repeated fourth or sixth hourly.Watch for tachyarrhythmias.
3. Dialysis is indicated in patients with severe renal impairment such as AKI or CKD.
    - It is one of the most effective methods of potassium removal.
    - Produces 1 mEq/L drop in serum K^+ after one hour.

Chapter

41

Hypokalemia

It is defined as serum potassium concentration of <3.5 mEq/L.

A total body K^+ deficit of 200–400 mEq is required to produce a 1 mEq decrease in plasma K^+

Causes of Hypokalemia

- Renal K^+ loss—accounts for most cases
  - Loop and thiazide diuretic use—cause alkalosis
  - Steroids, mineralocorticoid excess
  - Magnesium deficiency
  - Renal tubular acidosis (types 1 and 2)
  - Gitelman's syndrome and Barrter's syndrome
- Nonrenal K^+ loss—vomiting/nasogastric aspiration/diarrhea.
- Transcellular shift—due to alkalemia, insulin infusion, Beta 2 adrenergic agonists.
- Spurious—high numbers of metabolically active cells in the blood sample.

Clinical Features

Fatigue, myalgias, and muscular weakness or cramps of the lower extremities.

Constipation or frank paralytic ileus.

Life threatening—cardiac arrhythmias, ascending paralysis, respiratory muscle weakness

Investigations

Biochemistry

- Serum K, pH and HCO_3, plasma calcium, magnesium.
- If acidosis—DKA or RTA and diarrhoea.
- If alkalotic-vomiting, diuretic use and mineralocorticoid excess.
- Urine K >30 mEq/day suggests increased to establish renal loss, if cause is not evident.
- Urine chloride increased in diuretic therapy/Bartter's /Gitelman's syndrome.
- Transcellular gradient of K in urine >3, suggests renal loss.

ECG

- ST depression, T wave flattening, inversion, U wave appearance
- PR prolongation, atrial/ventricular tachyarrhythmias
- QT prolongation

Management

Mild hypokalemia (K—3 to 3.5 mEq/L)

- Potassium rich diet-like fruits, vegetables, spinach, nuts, tender coconut water, etc.
- Oral KCL with water or slow-release tablets
  - Oral KCl syrup: Daily doses range from 40 to 100 mEq given in 2 to 5 divided doses
  - Limit doses to 40 mEq per dose.
  - Commonly available oral preparations
  - KMac: Each 1 mL contains 2 mEq of K, Potklor syrup—each 15 mL contains 20 mEq of K.
  - Potassium sparing diuretics such as amiloride, spironolactone, eplerenone in patients with hypokalemia with renal loss.

Severe hypokalemia (K <2.5 mEq/L)

- Requires IV correction, especially if the patient is symptomatic.
- IV correction through a peripheral vein— at max 10 mEq/h, more rapid corrections of 20–40 mEq/h will require a central venous catheter.
- IV potassium should be infused in a non-dextrose containing saline solution.
- Standard method—add 20 mEq of KCl in 100 mL NS and infuse over 1 hour.
- For patients with severe hypokalemia due to gastrointestinal or renal losses, the recommended rate of potassium administration is 10–20 mEq/hour.
- In patients with life threatening hypokalemia, up to 40 mEq/hour of potassium can be given.

If hypokalemia is persisting or refractory to K^+ replacement, hypomagnesemia should be suspected and treated if present.

Chapter

42

Hyponatremia

Definition

Sodium concentration in serum of <135 mEq/L

- Mild hyponatremia—130–134 mEq/L
- Moderate hyponatremia—120–129 mEq/L
- Severe hyponatremia—<120 mEq/L

Classification

Pseudohyponatremia

- Occurs in high concentration of solutes occupying plasma (triglycerides >1500 mg/dL or serum protein >10 g/dL or high blood glucose)
- Translocational—due to presence of effective solutes—glucose, mannitol, maltose—high serum osmolarity + low Na levels
- Methodology related–when flame spectrophotometry method is used—normal serum osmolarity + low Na levels.

Correction Formula

- Serum sodium is decreased by 1.6 mEq/L for every 100 mg/dL increase in plasma glucose.
- Serum sodium is decreased by 1 mEq/L for every 500 mg/dL increase in plasma triglycerides above 100 mg/dL.
- Serum sodium is decreased by 4 mEq/L for every 1 g/dL increase in protein above 8 g/dL.

True Hyponatremia

Classification

Classified based on serum osmolarity (normal level—280–295 mOsm/kg) into hypovolemic, euvolemic, and hypervolemic.

Causes of Hyponatremia

Hypovolemic hyponatremia	Euvolemic hyponatremia	Hypervolemic hyponatremia
Renal causes Diuretic induced (**thiazide** >> loop) Interstitial nephritis Recovering AKI Mineralocorticoid deficiency Osmotic diuresis due to ketonuria, glucosuria, bicarbonaturia **Nonrenal causes** Cerebral salt wasting syndrome Excessive vomiting, diarrhea Burns Pancreatitis Small bowel obstruction Rhabdomyolysis	Syndrome of inappropriate ADH secretion (SIADH) Hypothyroidism Primary adrenal insufficiency Primary polydipsia Beer potomania	Cirrhosis of liver Chronic kidney disease Nephrotic syndrome Congestive cardiac failure

SIADH

Barrter and Schwartz diagnostic criteria for SIADH

- Serum osmolarity <275 mOsm/kg
- Clinically euvolemic
- Serum sodium <135 mEq/L
- Urine sodium >40 mEq/L
- Urine osmolarity >100 mOsmol/kg

To be checked before diagnosis of SIADH

- Normal renal functions
- Normal thyroxine and cortisol
- Excluding use of diuretics
- No hypokalemia

Other supplemental features

- Serum uric acid <4 mg/dL
- Low urea (single digit)
- Failure to correct hyponatremia after normal saline infusion

Causes of SIADH

CNS	Drug induced	Pulmonary	Malignancy
Stroke Meningitis Encephalitis Brain abscess IC bleeds Tumors Carbamazepine, valproate	SSRI Vincristine (all AEDS except levetiracetam) Cyclophosphamide Cisplatin TCA Desmopressin	Pneumonia TB Lung abscess	Small cell carcinoma lung Oropharyngeal carcinomas

Clinical Features

Acute hyponatremia

Sodium level of 120–135 mEq/L

- Nausea, vomiting and generalized weakness
- Headache

Sodium level of <120 mEq/L

- Lethargy/seizures/coma

Chronic hyponatremia

Usually asymptomatic up to sodium level of 120 mEq/L below which they manifest as

- Fatigue/nausea/vomiting
- Confusion/lethargy/coma

Diagnostic work up

1. Serum sodium
2. Serum osmolality can be measured/calculated
   - Serum osmolality = $(2 \times \text{Na}) + \dfrac{\text{Glucose}}{18} + \dfrac{\text{Blood urea nitrogen}}{2.8}$
   - Triglycerides, RBS, total protein is also estimated to rule out pseudohyponatremia.
3. Urine osmolality—higher than serum in SIADH (but any value >100 mOsm/kg is sufficient), low in other causes.
4. Urea, creatinine, uric acid, TSH or T_4 and cortisol levels.
5. Urine sodium and volume status

Volume status	Urine sodium	Etiology
Hypovolemic	<20 mEq/L	GI/third space loss
Hypervolemic	<20 mEq/L	Cardiac failure
Hypovolemic	>20 mEq/L	Diuretic use, renal loss
Euvolemic	>20 mEq/L	SIADH
Hypervolemic	>20 mEq/L	CKD

Treatment

Calculate Sodium Deficit

- Total body water (TBW) = 0.6 × body weight in males,
  = 0.5 × body weight in females
- Sodium deficit is TBW × (desired sodium – actual)
- Adrogué Madias formula-gives the degree to which 1 L of any given solution will rise serum Na.

  $$\text{Increase in serum sodium} = \frac{(\text{Infusate sodium} - \text{serum sodium})}{[\text{Total body water (TBW)} + 1]}$$

Acute Hyponatremia (can be corrected fast)

Goal of therapy: Raising serum sodium by 4–6 mEq/L every few hours

Symptomatic patients (even mild symptoms)—first 6 hours

- 100 mL bolus of 3% saline over 10 minutes up to 3 times

OR

- 150 mL bolus of 3% saline over 20 minutes up to 3 times

Regular monitoring of sodium levels every 2 hours and determine need for further therapy

Chronic Hyponatremia (always corrected slowly)

Mild hyponatremia (130–134 mEq/L)

Discontinue offending drugs. No active treatment required if asymptomatic

- Fluid restriction to <800 mL per day in patients with SIADH
- Oral salt up to 15 grams/day

Moderate hyponatremia (120–129 mEq/L)

Goal of correction: 4–6 mEq/L per 24 hours. Not more than 8–10 mEq/L.
In addition to above measures, vaptans can be used

Vaptans

- Vaptans—oral tolvaptan—15 mg on day 1, and can be increased to 30–60 mg/day thereafter
- Caution: LFT must be normal
- Water consumption must be unrestricted

IV conivaptan—20 mg IV bolus over 30 mins followed by 20 mg over 1 day. Can be increased to 40 mg over one day if increase in sodium is <5 mEq/L
Vaptans may not be effective when Cr >2.5 mg/dL

IV hypertonic saline

If patient has altered sensorium, either 1.6 or 3% saline can be used

- 3% saline contains—513 mEq of sodium per liter
- 1.6% saline contains—272 mEq of sodium per liter

Severe hyponatremia (<120mEq/L)

- Start 3% saline infusion initially at 15–30 mL/hr (0.25 to 0.5 mL/kg/hr) and titrate according to the next sodium value regardless of volume status.
- Rate of correction: Not more than 8–10 mEq/day if chronic hyponatremia.
- Faster correction leads to osmotic demyelination syndrome (ODS), causing demyelination of pons, with quadriplegia and severe neurological deficits.
- Chronic hyponatremia is most prone for ODS, hence serum sodium has to be monitored 4th hourly. Especially in alcoholics, malnourished, and liver failure patients.
- After correction with hypertonic saline, Inj. frusemide 40 mg IV stat can be given.It will increase water excretion, and raise serum sodium.

Note:

It is always advisable to repeat sodium levels every 6 hours, and recalculate, as rise is unpredictable, and over correction may occur.

Subsequent treatment of chronic hyponatremia

- Hypertonic saline infusion should be discontinued for the day when desired sodium increase has been achieved.
- Extra salt can continue.
- Vaptans can be stopped after achieving normal sodium levels.
- Potassium correction—if there is associated hypokalemia.

Hypovolemic hyponatremia

- 0.9% saline contains 154 mEq of sodium per litre.
- Volume status of the patient is to be continuously assessed.
- Parameters, like blood pressure, heart, rate are to be monitored.

Hypervolemic hyponatremia

- Fluid restriction to <800 mL/day
- Loop diuretics IV
- Treatment of underlying cause

Chapter

43

Hypernatremia

Serum sodium is the proportion of sodium in total body water (TBW). If TBW is low, serum sodium is high.

Definition

Serum sodium >145 mEq/L

- Acute hypernatremia-hypernatremia <48 hours.
- Chronic hypernatremia-hypernatremia persists >48 hours.

Mechanisms of Hypernatremia

Either due to water loss or due to sodium retention.

Water Loss

- Gastrointestinal loss-osmotic diarrhea, vomiting
- Urinary loss
- Central or nephrogenic diabetes insipidus
  - Osmotic diuresis—mannitol administration, DKA, HONK
  - Adipsic diabetes insipidus—when both ADH secretion and thirst is impaired
- Skin—sweating
- Exercise, fever, increased temperatures
- Postpartum hypernatremia due to production of vasopressinase

Sodium Retention

Iatrogenic—administration of large volumes of isotonic saline (0.9% NS) or hypertonic NaCl or $NaHCO_3$.

Clinical Manifestations

Acute hypernatremia (very rare). Usually unmasking of DI in the setting of acute water loss.

- Clinical features (due to cerebral dehydration and osmotic demyelination)
  - Thirst, Lethargy, Weakness — initial symptoms
  - Irritability, dizziness, delirium

- Seizures] severe symptoms
- Coma]
- Rarely: Rupture of cerebral veins causing SAH and focal IC bleeds

Evaluation of Hypernatremia

Investigations—urine osmolality, serum osmolarity and serum sodium

- If urine osmolarity <300—central or nephrogenic diabetes insipidus. Can be proved by rise in urine osmolarity after ADH replacement .
- If urine osmolarity is between 300 and 800—could be osmotic diuresis or diabetes insipidus.
- If urine osmolarity is > 800—most likely due to dehydration (DI cannot be excluded). In case urine osmolarity comes back to normal after treatment but serum osmolarity is still high, it is due to partial DI.

Management

- Initial fluid replenishment
  - Total body water = 0.6 × body weight in kg in males (0.5 in females)
  - Desired total body water (TBW) = Total body water × $\frac{\text{current serum sodium}}{\text{ideal serum sodium.}}$

    For example, in a 50 kg man with sodium of 160 mEq/L

    Total body water (TBW) = 0.6 × 50 = 30 L

    Desired body water = 30 × 160/140 = 34/1 L
  - Water deficit = desired total body water – present total body water.

    Water deficit = 4.1L
  - **In chronic hypernatremia** – hypernatremia for more than 48 hours
    - 5% dextrose is used as choice of IV fluid at 1.35 mL/kg/hour 45% saline (half normal saline), can also be used, especially in diabetics
    - Hypernatremic patients who are also hypovolemic will also require isotonic fluids.
    - Oral or ryle's tube free water (100 to 150 mL 2nd hourly) can also be given in stable patients
    - Repeat sodium levels every 4 hours, till target is reached .
    - **Account for ongoing losses of water**
    - **Goal of sodium reduction: 10 mEq/day.** Not >12 mEq per day. Faster correction can lead to cerebral edema.
  - In acute hypernatremia (rare-seen in DI with water loss)
    - Seen in diabetes insipidus.
    - 5% dextrose is started at 3–6 mL/kg/hour
    - At 145 mEq/L , reduce to fluid rate to 1 mL/kg/hr till 140 mEq/L
    - Serum sodium is repeated Q_2H.
    - Sodium levels are decreased at 1–2 mEq per hour and brought down to normal within 1 day.

- Patients with central diabetes insipidus will also require desmopressin therapy.
- In case of hyperglycemia, drip rate can be reduced, or 2.5% dextrose can be used.

- Hypernatremia due to correction of hyperglycemia
  - Correction of hyperglycemia and hypovolemia in patients with DKA or HHS can cause hypernatremia due to osmotic shift of water from ECF to cells.
  - It is managed in the same way how chronic hypernatremia is managed.
- Patients with hypovolemia or superadded hypokalemia

In case there is dehydration with hypokalemia, free water can be given along with the addition of a second IV fluid for potassium correction.

Chapter

44

Hypocalcemia

Serum calcium levels less than 8.4 mg/dL is considered as hypocalcemia.

Pseudohypocalcemia

- Most labs check total serum calcium rather than the metabolically active ionized calcium
- Calcium is bound to serum albumin and hence the albumin levels can affect the calcium.
- Add 0.8 mg/dL for every 1 gm fall in serum albumin.
  corrected calcium = 0.8 × (4-serum albumin) + measured calcium
  This is a rough calculation, and may not be accurate. May need to ionised calcium, if patient is in ICU.

Causes of Hypocalcemia

A. With low PTH
   - Postsurgery—thyroidectomy, parathyroidectomy and radical neck dissection.
   - Autoimmune hypoparathyroidism

B. With high PTH—secondary hyperparathyroidism
   - Vitamin D deficiency
   - Renal disease—CKD
   - Tumor lysis
   - Pancreatitis
   - Acute respiratory alkalosis
   - Hyperphosphatemia

C. Other causes
   - Drugs, e.g. bisphosphonates, calcitonin, denosumab, cinacalcet, etc.
   - Hypomagnesemia
   - Sepsis

Clinical Features

- Tetany—characterised by neuromuscular irritability. Symptoms start with perioral and acral paresthesia.
- Myalgia and muscle cramps, e.g. carpal spasm, laryngismus stridulus. Fasciculations and hyperreflexia can occur.

- Seizures
- Psychiatric problems—emotional instability, anxiety, depression and psychosis.

Signs

- Trousseau's sign—inflation of the sphygmomanometer >20 mmHg above systolic blood pressure for 3 minutes will cause carpal spasm of hand
- Chvostek's sign—contraction of the ipsilateral facial muscles that can be elicited by tapping on the facial nerve just anterior to the ear.

Investigations

- Serum calcium, phosphorus, alkaline phosphatase, magnesium and albumin
- Vit D
- PTH
- ECG—prolonged QT interval, due to prolonged ST segment, bradycardia, with normal T waves, complete heart block.

Management

Severe acute hypocalcemia

The following are indications for IV correction of hypocalcemia:

- Symptoms such as carpopedal spasm, tetany and seizures
- Prolonged QT interval
- Asymptomatic acute hypocalcemia such as postoperative patients with calcium less than 7.5 mg/dL

Initially IV calcium 2 g (20 mL) of calcium gluconate 10% over 15 minutes—to be diluted in 50–100 mL of 5% dextrose or NS.

(1 gram (10 mL) of calcium gluconate contains 90 mg of elemental calcium)

Persistent hypocalcemia

- Initial correction followed by infusion. Add 6 to 8 ampules of calcium gluconate (each ampoule – 90 mg of elemental calcium) in 500 mL 5% dextrose to be given over 6 to 8 hours. Approx 1–3 mg of elemental calcium/kg/hr
- Monitor every 6 hours, till calcium normalises.
- Overlap with oral calcium as given below.

Mild or Chronic Hypocalcemia

- Oral supplementation of calcium: 1 to 2 g of elemental calcium per day. Calcium content is 40% in carbonate, 36% in chloride, 8% gluconate
- Vitamin D supplementation is required in patients with hypoparathyroidism, vitamin D deficiency, CKD and CLD. Vitamin D or its metabolites (calcitriol, calcidiol) can be used.
- Calcitriol dose 0.25 to 2 micrograms/day. Uptitrated weekly to target.

Other Measures

- Concurrent hypomagnesemia should be looked for and corrected: Add 2 gm IV of magnesium sulphate over 15 minutes if renal function is normal.

Chapter

45

Hypercalcemia

Definition

Serum calcium of more than 11 mg/dL.

- Most labs check total serum calcium, not metabolically active ionized calcium.
- Calcium is bound to serum albumin and hence the albumin levels can affect the calcium.
- Add 0.8 mg/dL for every 1 gm fall in serum albumin.

Causes

Normal or elevated PTH
• Primary hyperparathyroidism
• Tertiary hyperparathyroidism
• Familial hypocalciuric hypercalcemia
With low PTH levels
• Malignancy
• Excess vitamin D
• Thyrotoxicosis/Sarcoidosis/TB
• Prolonged immobilization
• Milk alkali syndrome
• Drugs—Thiazides

Clinical Features

- Mild hypercalcemia (<11.5 mg/dL)—asymptomatic/nonspecific symptoms
- Moderate hypercalcemia–(11.5 to 14 mg/dL).
- Severe hypercalcemia (>14 mg/dL)

Chronic hypercalcaemia—well tolerated
acute rise—may cause marked symptoms

Symptoms and Signs

Renal: Polyuria, polydipsia and nephrolithiasis

Gastrointestinal: Anorexia, nausea, vomiting, constipation, pancreatitis and peptic ulcer disease.

Musculoskeletal: Weakness or pathological fractures and osteoporosis.

Neuropsychiatric: Decreased concentration, confusion, personality changes, seizure and coma.

Cardiovascular: Hypertension—deposition of calcium in the vessel wall.

Most hyperparathyroidism is mild hypercalcemia, and hence asymptomatic. Hypercalcemia due to malignancy is usually symptomatic, as levels are high.

Management

Investigations

- Serum calcium, phosphorous, alkaline phosphatase, and albumin
- Vitamin D levels
- PTH or PTHrP if suspecting malignancy.
- ECG—short QT interval
- Investigations for cause: Malignancy, sarcoidosis, etc.

Important: If serum calcium is high, and PTH is normal, it is still hyperparathyroidism. This is because, PTH is inappropriately high, and may fluctuate.

Treatment

Mild hypercalcemia

- Usually do not require immediate treatment.
- Avoid thiazides and unnecessary calcium supplementation.
- Avoid volume depletion and ensure adequate hydration.

Moderate hypercalcemia

- If asymptomatic or chronic hypercalcemia may not require immediate treatment
- If symptomatic or acute hypercalcemia, immediate management should be initiated as described below.

Severe hypercalcemia

Immediate therapy includes:

- Volume expansion with isotonic saline at an initial rate of 200 to 300 mL/hour.
- May require up to 4–6 L in the first 24 hr.
- Loop diuretics should be started only after adequate volume expansion, e.g. Inj frusemide 40 mg IV can be given every 1 liter of fluids.
- Calcitonin (fastest acting drug 4 hours) causes reduction in the bone resorption.
  - Given IM or SC–4 IU/kg. Can be repeated every 6 to 12 hours.
  - Patients may develop tachyphylaxis to calcitonin after 24 to 48 hours.
- Bisphosphonates cause reduction in hypercalcemia by being taken up by osteoclasts and results in apoptosis and causes reduction in bone resorption. Will act from 2–4 days.
  - Zoledronic acid—4 mg IV over 15 minutes (in 100 mL saline). Not recommended below creatinine clearance of 30 mL/min.
  - Pamidronate—60 to 90 mg IV over 2 hours

- Denosumab—human monoclonal antibody to RANKL. It inhibits osteoclast formation, decreases bone resorption.
  - It is given subcutaneously as a single dose of 120 mg. Can be repeated in same dose every week for 4 weeks, and then monthly, in malignancy induced hypercalcemia .
- Steroids: Useful in Vit D mediated hypercalcemia—sarcoidosis and lymphoma.

  Dexamethasone 4 mg IV 8th hourly or IV hydrocortisone 100–300 mg daily or prednisolone 40–60 mg daily for 3–7 days.
- Cinacalcet: Reduces PTH secretion by acting on CaSR (calcium sensing receptor) used in parathyroid cancer, primary hyperparathyroidism, secondary hyperparathyroidism in renal failure.
  - Dose: 30–90 mg daily orally. Increased weekly from 30 mg daily.
- Dialysis—should be considered when:
  - Serum calcium >18 mg/dL.
  - Neurological symptoms.
  - Complicated with renal failure.
  - Failure of other treatment options to reduce the serum calcium levels.

Chapter

46

Hypomagnesemia

Definition

- Serum magnesium <1.8 mg/dL
  Often accompanied by depletion of potassium, phosphate, and calcium .

Etiology

- Decreased intake or absorption:
  - Malnutrition
- Increased loss
  - GI loss: Diarrhea, laxative abuse, vomiting and nasogastric suction.
  - Renal loss: Drugs diuretics, loop diuretics, thiazide diuretics, antibiotics-aminoglycosides and amphotericin B
  - Skin loss:
  - Burns
- Redistribution from extracellular to intracellular compartment
  - Refeeding syndrome
- Pseudohypomagnesemia:
  - Collection of blood in potassium EDTA
  - Hypoalbuminemia

Clinical features

- Asymptomatic until serum magnesium levels <1.2 mg/dL.
- Mild to moderate hypomagnesemia—nausea/vomiting/fatigue
- Moderate to severe hypomagnesemia
  - Neuromuscular and CNS:
    - Tingling and numbness
    - Muscle weakness and cramps
    - Agitation, depression, psychosis
    - Seizures/coma
  - Cardiac:
    - Atrial and ventricular arrhythmias (including torsades de pointes)

Presenting features may overlap with features of electrolyte abnormalities which are commonly associated with hypomagnesemia, such as, hypokalemia and hypocalcemia

Investigations

- Serum magnesium levels:
  - Mild to moderate hypomagnesemia: 1 to 1.6 mg/dL
  - Severe hypomagnesemia: <1 mg/dL
- Metabolic profile, including Urea, creatinine, sodium, potassium, chloride, bicarbonate, calcium and blood glucose levels

Management

- Severe or symptomatic hypomagnesemia:
  - 1 g of magnesium sulfate contains 4 mmol (or 8 mEq) of elemental magnesium
  - Treatment goal: Serum magnesium > 1mg/dL
    - In cases of hemodynamic instability, life-threatening arrhythmias such as torsades de pointes, or if the patient is actively seizing:
      - 1 to 2 g magnesium sulfate IV diluted in water, given slowly, over 15 minutes is administered
      - Repeat if necessary in 5 to 15 minutes
      - Thereafter, begin magnesium infusion as given below.
      - Check loss of deep tendon reflexes to detect hypermagnesemia.

  Hemodynamically stable:

  - 8 to 12 g of magnesium sulfate IV given in the initial 24 hours
  - 1 to 2 grams of magnesium sulfate in 50 to 100 mL of 5% dextrose given initially over 5 to 60 minutes followed by an infusion
  - Infusion—4 to 8 grams given slowly over 12–24 hours
  - Followed by 4 to 6 g/day for 3 or 4 days to replete body stores
  - Infusion rate **should not exceed 2 g/hour**
  - In patients with renal insufficiency, **25–50%** of the initial dose is given
- For mild or moderate asymptomatic hypomagnesemia
  - Oral replacement: 120 to 336 mg elemental magnesium PO in divided doses, daily for normal renal function.
  - Adverse effect: Diarrhea
  - If refractory or intolerant: Amiloride and triamterene, to decrease renal loss
  - Correction of concurrent electrolyte abnormalities

Monitoring during infusion

- Monitor blood pressure, respiratory rate, and deep tendon reflexes
  - Stop administration if signs of hypermagnesemia or magnesium intoxication such as hypotension, bradypnea or hyporeflexia develop.
- Monitor serum magnesium levels, at least twice daily.
- ECG monitoring is recommended for patients treated with high doses, rapid doses, and in the elderly.

Chapter

47

Hypophosphatemia

Etiology

Reduced renal tubular phosphate reabsorption

1. Primary hyperparathyroidism
2. Vitamin D deficiency
3. Alcoholism
4. Hypomagnesemia
5. Fanconi's syndrome: Tenofovir, cisplatin, ifosfamide, foscarnet, rapamycin

Impaired intestinal absorption

1. Chronic diarrhea/aluminium containing antacids

Intracellular shift of phosphorous

1. Acute respiratory alkalosis
2. Recovery from starvation—refeeding

Accelerated net bone formation

1. After parathyroidectomy—hungry bone syndrome
2. Osteoblastic metastasis

Clinical Features

Depends on severity/chronicity

Overt symptoms: Serum phosphate levels are <2 mg/dL

- Nervous system: Lethargy, confusion, paraesthesia, generalized or ascending paralysis, cardiopulmonary system—ventricular arrhythmias
- Skeletal and smooth muscle—aches and pains, proximal myopathy, rhabdomyolysis if severe (<1 mg/dL)
- Hematological—hemolysis
- Severe symptoms like seizures, coma

EVALUATION

1. Normal serum phosphate levels (2.5–4.5 mg/dL)
2. Serum calcium, ALP, urea/creatinine
3. Vitamin D levels decreased (calcium low, phosphorous low)
4. PTH increased (calcium increase, phosphorus low)

5. 24-hour urine phosphorus or fractional excretion of phosphate (>100 mg/5% indicates a renal phosphate wasting)

Treatment

In asymptomatic: Oral replacement.

Treat underlying cause.

In symptomatic patients

a. 1–1.9 mg/dL treat orally
b. <1 mg/dL—intravenous correction
c. Switch to oral correction when more than 1.5 mg/dL

INTRAVENOUS THERAPY

Serum phosphate <1.25 mg/dL

Infusion of 0.25 to 0.50 mmol/kg given over 8–12 hours (max up to 80 mmol)

Serum phosphate >1.25 mg/dL

Infusion of 0.08 to 0.24 mmol/kg over six hours (max up to 30 mmol)

Preparation—Potphos (1 mL gives 93 mg or 3 mmol of elemental phosphate)

10 mL in 40 mL NS over 8 hours. Monitor K^+ and phosphorus levels.

Note

1. Monitor serum phosphate levels every 6 hours
2. Check serum calcium (correct hypocalcemia before intravenous therapy and reduce the dose by 50% in hypercalcemia).
3. Renal function (reduce dose by 50% if serum creatinine >2.5 mg/dL)

ORAL THERAPY

<1.5 mg/dL, give 1.3 mmol/kg of elemental phosphorus (max 100 mmol) in three to four divided doses over 24 hours.

>1.5 mg/dL, give 1 mmol/kg of elemental phosphorus (max 80 mmol) in three to four divided doses over 24 hours.

Available preparation—addphos; each sachet contains 16.1 mmol of elemental phosphate.

Section

6

Endocrinology

Chapter

48

Diabetic Ketoacidosis (DKA)

It is a serious, acute complication of diabetic mellitus (DM).

Definition

1. Hyperglycemia—the serum glucose levels are usually between 250 and 500 mg/dL. It can even exceed 800 mg/dL.
2. High anion gap acidosis—anion gap > 20, pH < 7.3 and bicarbonate < 15 mmol/L.
3. Ketosis—positive serum or urine ketones.

Clinical Features

Symptoms	Physical findings
• Nausea/vomiting • Thirst/polyuria • Abdominal pain • Shortness of breath **Precipitating events** • Inadequate or missed insulin (type 1 DM) • Infection • Infarction (cerebral, coronary) • Drugs (cocaine) • Pregnancy • Unprovoked ketosis occurs in type 1 DM	• Tachycardia • Dehydration/hypotension • Tachypnea/Kussmaul respirations/ respiratory distress • Abdominal tenderness (may resemble acute pancreatitis or surgical abdomen) • Lethargy/obtundation/cerebral edema/ possibly coma

Investigations

- Serum glucose >250 mg/dL
- Serum sodium will be falsely low in view of the high sugars (1.6 mmol/L reduction in serum sodium for each 100 mg/dL rise in the serum glucose)
- Serum potassium at presentation may be mildly elevated, secondary to the acidosis and volume depletion, in spite of reduced total K
- Anion gap calculation = Serum Na – (serum HCO_3^- + serum chloride). DKA will have a high anion gap in view of ketone formation.
- Serum creatinine—might be elevated, reflecting the reduced intravascular volume.
- TC increased of >25,000 cells/mL suggests infection
- Urinalysis and urine ketones by dipstick positive
- Plasma osmolality will be increased in view of the hyperglycemia—300 to 330 mOsm/L

- Serum ketones positive—not commonly done
- Urine ketones—positive
- Arterial blood gas—pH low., serum bicarbonate <13 mEq/L
- Serum amylase and lipase if pancreatitis is suspected, precipitating DKA.
- Amylase can be high without pancreatitis also in DKA
- Investigations to identify the precipitating cause of the DKA like infections, should also be sent
- Electrocardiogram

Treatment

Principles include correction of:

1. Fluid
2. Hyperglycemia
3. Electrolyte imbalance
4. Acidosis
5. Management of infection

Fluid Management

- In DKA, patients have a deficit of about 6 to 8 liters in the extracellular compartment. This needs to be corrected with IV fluids and oral intake wherever possible.
- Strict input output chart required
    - To start with IV 0.9% NS which is to be given as:
        - 1 litre in the first half hour
        - 1 litre in the next 1 hour
        - 1 litre in the next 2 hours
- The rate can be titrated based on the amount of dehydration, age, and cardiac status of the patient.
- If the serum sodium is more than 155 mEq/L, 0.45 normal saline can be used at 250 to 500 mL/hr.
- Once sugars drop to less than 200 mg/dL, then change to 5% dextrose to avoid hypoglycemia, and correct intracellular dehydration.

Hyperglycemia

- Regular insulin to be used.
- Initial IV bolus dose of 0.1 units/kg to be given
- This is followed by an infusion of regular insulin at 0.1 units/kg/hour. It is prepared by adding 1 mL insulin (40 units) in 39 mL NS and then given as an infusion.
- GRBS to be done hourly as shown in DKA chart
- Blood glucose should fall by 50 to 100 mg per hour.
- Do not allow hypoglycemia: It will cause rebound increase in sugars due to counter regulatory hormones
- When serum glucose levels reach 200 mg/dL, the rate of infusion can be reduced to 0.05 units/kg/hour.
- **The end point of insulin therapy is the resolution of ketosis and closure of anion gap.** For this insulin may have to be continued in spite of sugar falling below

200 mg/dL. At this point 5% D solution has to be started and insulin continued till ketosis resolves.

- The blood glucose should be maintained at around 150 to 200 mg/dL until the DKA resolves.
- Change to basal insulin, along with subcutaneous insulin with every meal once the patient starts to take orally.
- There should be an overlap of 2–4 hours of infusion insulin, during switching over to subcutaneous insulin, otherwise sugars may increase.

Electrolyte Imbalance

Potassium correction:

- Serum K <3.3 mEq/L—hold insulin and start IV K at 40 mEq/L
- If serum K is 3.5–5.5 mEq/L, add 20 to 30 mEq of K in each litre of IV fluids to maintain serum K between 4 and 5 mEq/L.
- If >5.5 mEq/L no correction required only regular monitoring
- Serum urea and creatine should be monitored.

Ketosis Monitoring

- The predominant ketones are beta hydroxy butyric acid (BHBA) in DKA, but urine ketones detect acetoacetate.
- BHBA is converted to acetoacetate with improving perfusion.
- So ketones can falsely increase when hydration improves in DKA.

Acidosis

- Acidosis should only be corrected with IV sodium bicarbonate if pH is <6.9.

Infection

- Most DKAs are precipitated by an infection and these should be treated accordingly .

Monitoring

- GRBS should be checked hourly until resolution of DKA
- Criteria for resolution of ketosis:
  - Blood sugar <200 mg/dL
  - pH >7.3
  - HCO_3 >15 mEq/dL
  - Closure of anion gap
  - Patient able to eat normally
- Renal function tests, VBG can be checked every 4 hours
- Urine ketones can be checked every 6 hours for resolution

Complications

- Lactic acidosis
- Cerebral edema—common in children.

Diabetic Ketoacidosis (DKA) Monitoring Chart (Flowchart 48.1)

Flowchart 48.1: DKA chart should be maintained for easy monitoring of the various parameters.

Date: Patient details

Time	GRBS	Insulin (Basal)	Insulin (bolus)	Urine	IV fluid (rate, type)	Oral intake	Output	Pulse/ BP	pH	HCO_3	Na/K/ Cl	Anion gap
0600												
0700												
0800												
0900												
1000												
1100												
1200												
1300												
1400												
1500												
1600												
1700												
1800												
1900												
2000												
2100												
2200												
2300												
0000												
0100												
0200												
0300												
0400												
0500												

Hyperglycemic Hyperosmolar State

Insulin levels enough to prevent lipolysis, not enough to prevent hyperglycemia

Definition

- Severe hyperglycemia—>600 mg/dL
- Hyperosmolality—serum osmolality >320 mOsm/kg (if less than 320 mOsm/kg, look for another cause for altered sensorium)
- Dehydration
- No ketones or acidosis

(It was previously referred to as HONK (hyperosmolar non ketotic coma), which is no longer used as the presentation with coma is not common.)

Clinical Features

- Elderly individual with type 2 DM
- Precipitated by stress: Myocardial infarction/pneumonia/stroke

- Reduced fluid intake
- Confusion and lethargy.
- O/E dehydration including hypotension, tachycardia and altered mental status.
- No signs of acidosis

Management of HHS

- Correction of fluid and electrolyte deficit
- Give adequate fluid replacement—up to 10 litres may be required in some patients
- Start fluid replacement with 0.9% NS which can be changed to 0.45%NS if the serum osmolality increases in spite of positive fluid balance.
- 250–500 mL/hr speed of correction based on patient's cardiac and renal status in addition to hypotension
- Treat till patient becomes arousable, and osmolality normalises
- Insulin infusion should be initiated at 0.05 U/kg/hr.
- Treat coexisting conditions
- Give prophylactic anticoagulation in dehydrated patients prone to thrombosis.
- Treat the underlying condition that precipitated the HHS
- The rest of the management is similar to DKA

EUGLYCEMIC KETOACIDOSIS

Ketosis occurs in the context of starvation and dehydration, with ketone in urine, but normal sugars.

Causes

- Starvation in pregnancy or otherwise
- Acute conditions: Surgery, infection and trauma
- Alcohol
- Insulin withdrawal
- SGLT2 inhibitors—canagliflozin, empagliflozin in diabetic patients

Clinical Features

- Acidosis: Tachypnea and weakness
- Dehydration, hypotension and altered sensorium
- No polyuria and polydipsia of hyperglycemia

Investigations

Sugar 250 mg/dL, pH <7.3, HCO_3^- <18 mEq/L, ketones in urine, hypomagnesemia, hypophosphatemia of starvation.

Treatment

- IV fluids at 200 mL/hr NS or Ringer's lactate till dehydration settles
- Insulin to be started at DKA dose: 5% dextrose may be needed as sugar levels are not high, as insulin is needed till acidosis resolves.
- Treat precipitating factor

Chapter

49

Hypoglycemia

- Blood glucose levels of less than 70 mg/dL is known as hypoglycemia.
- Documented by the Whipple's triad:
  - Symptoms consistent with hypoglycemia
  - Low plasma glucose levels
  - Relief of symptoms after the plasma glucose levels are raised

Hypoglycemia alert value (level 1)	≤70 mg/dL (3.9 mmol/L)	Sufficiently low for treatment with fast-acting carbohydrate and dose adjustment of glucose-lowering therapy
Clinically significant hypoglycemia (level 2)	<54 mg/dL (3.0 mmol/L)	Sufficiently low to indicate serious, clinically important hypoglycemia
Severe hypoglycemia (level 3)	No specific glucose threshold	Hypoglycemia associated with severe cognitive impairment requiring external assistance for recovery

Causes

Ill or medicated patients
1. Drugs • Insulin or OHAs—sulphonylurea (SU), non-SU like repaglinide • Alcohol • Quinine/artemisinin • Trimethoprim/gatifloxacin • Phenytoin/NSAIDs
2. Critical illness • Hepatic or renal failure • Sepsis
3. Hormone deficiency • Cortisol—Addisons • Growth hormone • Glucagon
4. Non-islet cell tumors, hepatoma and carcinoid

Contd.

Contd.

Seemingly well individuals
1. Endogenous hyperinsulinism • Insulinoma • Insulin autoimmune hypoglycemia
2. Unusual exercise in diabetic, or missed meals, or wrong dose of insulin
3. Malicious hypoglycemia/factitious hypoglycemia

Pseudohypoglycemia

Falsely low glucometer readings can occur when patient is in circulatory shock, in ICU settings. Use arterial/venous blood in these settings.

Lab sugars can be falsely low in:

- Leukemias, polycythemia vera—due to glycolysis by the blood cells. Also sugar may be low, if the sample is not processed/refrigerated within 2 hours.
- Hypertriglyceridemia/paraproteinemias can also cause falsely low sugar.

Clinical picture: History

Type 1 and type 2 diabetes patient with missed meal, excess dose of insulin/SU, new onset renal failure, or hypothyroidism.

Note

New onset renal failure is one of the important causes of hypoglycemia without any change in diet or dose of drugs.

Symptoms

- Adrenergic (<70 mg/dL)— sudden profuse sweating, giddiness, tremors, palpitations, anxiety and hunger.
- Neuroglycopenic (<40 mg/dL)—drowsiness, altered sensorium, delirium, convulsions, coma, focal neurological deficits (hemiplegia)—rarely.
- Patients with autonomic neuropathy due to diabetes,especially in elderly/on beta blockers, may not have sympathetic warning symptoms, and may present with neuroglycopenia directly.
- Type 1 DM with recurrent hypoglycemia may have functional autonomic failure (hypoglycemia associated autonomic failure: HAAF). They also may present without sympathetic symptoms, with neuroglycopenia only.

Investigations

- Due to its varied clinical presentation, blood sugar levels should be checked in any patient that is brought in delirium or comatose state, especially in diabetics, alcoholics and individuals with extensive liver disease.
- By glucometer in emergency/confirm by lab sugar
- LFT, RFT.
- Fasting C-peptid and FBS for insulinoma
- Cortisol and thyroid function tests if needed

Management

- Stop or withhold insulin and all OHAs
- Administer glucose:
  - Oral glucose—in patients who are conscious. Plain sugars or sugar solutions/sugar rich food such as chocolates should be given.
  - If unconscious, IV glucose:
    - 50 mL of 50% dextrose as an IV bolus recheck sugar by glucometer after 15 minutes, to decide further treatment. This can be repeated if necessary
    - 10% dextrose IV infusion can be continued for 24 hours. This is for avoiding hypoglycemia that could present later due to long acting insulins or OHAs.
    - The patient can also be asked to take a meal after regaining consciousness.
- Glucagon (IV access is not available or resistant to IV dextrose):
  - Dose—1 mg IM/SC stat
  - The dose can be repeated in 10 minutes if required
- In case of prolonged hypoglycemic coma with convulsions:
  - Inj mannitol (20%) 200 mL IV stat for the cerebral edema
  - Inj dexamethasone 4 mg IV q8 h for edema and the hypoglycemia
- Cause for hypoglycemia should be evaluated. The most common cause for hypoglycemia in diabetic patients are overdosage of medication, intercurrent infections and renal failure.
- Adjust the dose of OHAs and insulin if necessary
- Counsel and educate patients and family members on how to identify and treat future hypoglycemic episodes at home.
- Patient should be instructed to always carry some form of oral glucose with them at all times.

Chapter

50

Myxedema Coma

Definition

Severe hypothyroidism leading to decreased mental function, hypothermia and signs of slowing down of organ systems.

Risk Factors

- Long standing untreated hypothyroidism
- Acute stressful event in poorly controlled hypothyroidism such as
  - Surgery
  - Infection
  - Extreme cold exposure
  - Myocardial infarction
- Drug induced—amiodarone, opioids and lithium
- Unusual causes of hypothyroidism
  - Postablative/postsurgical
  - Autoimmune thyroiditis

Clinical Features

- Neurological manifestations-
  - Confusion/lethargy/coma (less frequent)
  - Seizures/status epilepticus-likely due to secondary cause (hyponatremia, hypoglycemia)
- Hyponatremia—most common electrolyte imbalance
  - Usually due to inappropriate excess vasopressin secretion
  - Due to adrenal insufficiency(hypothyroidism associated with hypoadrenalism)
- Hypothermia
- Hypoglycemia
- Hypoventilation
  - Central respiratory depression
  - Obstructive sleep apnea due to large tongue
- Cardiac manifestations
  - Bradycardia
  - Hypotension(severe)
  - Pericardial effusion

Lab Diagnosis

- Low total T4/free T4
- High TSH—primary hypothyroidism—most common
- TSH can be normal or low—central hypothyroidism (uncommon)
- Low cortisol—to look for associated primary adrenal insufficiency
- Hyponatremia, hypothermia and hypercarbia.

Treatment

- Thyroid hormone replacement
  - As IV thyroxine is not available, we give thyroxine: 100 micrograms tid, through ryle's tube (split dose to avoid surge in thyroxine levels causing arrhythmia/MI)
  - If IV thyroxine is available a single bolus dose of 200–400 μg IV can be given followed by an oral dose of 1.6 μg/kg/d
  - Recheck T4 levels after 48 hours and adjust
  - Hydrocortisone 100 mg IV 8th hourly should be administered until adrenal insufficiency is ruled out
- Supportive measures
  - Correction of hypotension with fluids and vasopressors
  - Treat infection
  - Treatment of hyponatremia and hypoglycemia
  - Rewarming blankets
  - Mechanical ventilation if indicated

Prognosis

Mortality rate is 30–50%.
Poor prognosis factors:

- Older age
- Cardiac complications
- Reduced consciousness
- Mechanical ventilation
- Persistent hypothermia
- Sepsis

Chapter

51

Thyroid Storm

- Rare, life-threatening condition (mortality—10%)
- Severe clinical manifestations of thyrotoxicosis
- Patients with longstanding untreated hyperthyroidism

Precipitating Factors

- Thyroid/non-thyroidal surgery
- Infection
- Discontinuation of anti-thyroid drugs
- Radioiodine therapy for Graves' disease—rarely

Clinical Features

Exaggeration of usual symptoms of hyperthyroidism

- Cardiovascular
  - Tachycardia—>140/m, atrial fibrillation
  - Symptoms of congestive heart failure—in elderly
  - Hypotension, death from cardiovascular collapse
- Hyperpyrexia (104°–106°F)
- Psychiatric—altered mentation—agitation, anxiety, delirium, psychosis, stupor, coma
- Gastrointestinal—vomiting, diarrhea, abdominal pain and hepatic failure with jaundice
- Goitre, ophthalmopathy, lid lag, hand tremor, warm and moist skin

Laboratory Findings

- Low TSH, high total or free T4/T3
- Mild hyperglycemia (secondary to catecholamine release)
- Mild hypercalcemia (hemoconcentration and enhanced bone resorption)
- Abnormal LFT including bilirubin rise; liver enzymes up to 3 times of normal
- Leukocytosis/leukopenia

Management

- **Beta-blockers** (control symptoms and signs of sympathetic overactivity)
  - Oral Propranolol—60–80 mg q4 h – q6 h, based on HR and BP, or
  - IV propranolol 0.5–1 mg over 10 min followed by 1–2 mg over 10 min every 4 hours.

- Antithyroid drugs—thionamides to block new hormone synthesis
    - Propylthiouracil (PTU) loading dose 500–1000 mg followed by 250 mg q4 h (preferred—as it has additional inhibition of peripheral T4–T3 conversion) through Ryle's tube
    - Carbimazole 40–60 mg daily
- **Iodine**—to block new hormone synthesis (Wolff-Chaikoff effect)
    - **One hour after first dose of thionamide** (to prevent iodine from being used as a substrate for new hormone synthesis)
    - Saturated solution of potassium iodide—5 drops q6 h
    - Lugol's solution—10 drops q8 h
- **Glucocorticoids**—reduces T4 to T3 conversion
    - Promotes vasomotor stability
    - Hydrocortisone 200 mg IV stat, 100 mg IV q8 h, or
    - Dexamethasone 2 mg q 6th hourly
- **Bile acid sequestrants**
    - Reduces enterohepatic recycling of thyroid hormones
    - Cholestyramine – 4 g q6 h
- **Treat infection—most important precipitating cause**
- Supportive care: ICU care and monitoring
    - Appropriate fluid management—fluids (in dehydrated patients) versus diuretics (in patients with cardiac failure)
    - Paracetamol—for hyperpyrexia (avoid aspirin—as it can increase FT4 and FT3 by interfering with protein binding)
    - Plasmapheresis—removes cytokines, antibodies, thyroid hormone in plasma
- Definitive management of underlying cause for hyperthyroidism.

Chapter

52

Addisonian Crisis

- Refers to acute adrenal cortical insufficiency
- Potentially fatal, if not recognised and promptly managed

Causes

A: Iatrogenic
  - Abrupt withdrawal of exogenous steroids

B: Primary—all hormones of adrenal cortex deficient
  - Autoimmune adrenalitis
  - Adrenal tuberculosis
  - Adrenal infections, with adrenal hemorrhage due to DIC (Waterhouse-Friderichson's syndrome
  - Adrenal metastasis (from a distant primary, like lung)

C: Secondary—glucocorticoid and sex hormone deficiency
  - HPA axis failure

Precipitating Factors

- Infections
- Surgery
- Sudden tapering of exogenous steroids
- Initiation of thyroid hormone supplementation without concomitant steroid supplements in secondary adrenal insufficiency.

Symptoms and Signs

- Fatigue and weakness
- Postural giddiness, hypotension, with marked postural drop
- Abdominal pain, nausea and vomiting
- Weight loss (in case of acute of chronic), anorexia
- Myalgia, joint pain and fever
- Lethargy, decreased responsiveness, stupor and coma
- Hyperpigmentation (in case of primary adrenal insufficiency)

Diagnosis

- Low serum cortisol/inappropriately normal cortisol in conditions of stress
  - Random cortisol—may not be reliable

  - **low 8 am cortisol** (<3 μg/dL)—very suggestive; do not delay treatment, for sending tests
- **Hyponatremia with hyperkalemia** (in primary insufficiency, due to mineralocorticoid deficiency). Not seen in exogenous steroid withdrawal, as mineralocorticoid action is intact.
- Normocytic normochromic anemia, lymphocytosis and **eosinophilia**
- **Hypoglycemia**
- Metabolic acidosis (secondary to RTA), RFT abnormal

Special tests

- ACTH— >2 times upper limit of normal in primary, decreased in iatrogenic and secondary
- **Short cosyntropin test:**
  - To do plasma cortisol 30–60 min after 250 μg Cosyntropin (IV/IM) a rise of <9 μg/dL, or total of < 18 μg/dL—diagnostic of primary adrenal insufficiency.
- TSH, FT4, testosterone levels—to rule out hypopituitarism
- Adrenal imaging—USG abdomen/CECT abdomen
- MRI pituitary—in case secondary adrenal insufficiency is suspected

Treatment

- Fluid resuscitation—IV fluids NS or DNS (if hypoglycemia)—1 litre in first hour and 2 to 6 litres over 24 hours – then modify based on fluid status/response
- Hydrocortisone IV – 100 mg IV stat, followed by 100 mg IV q4 h/q6 h till crisis improves. Continue at 50–100 mg q 6th hourly, till patient is able to take orally.
- Maintenance oral steroids, after tiding over acute crisis
- Prednisolone 5 to 7.5 mg/day, either as single dose morning, or 5 mg and 2.5 mg morning and evening respectively as maintenance replacement.
  - To give extra doses during intercurrent illness/stress
- Maintenance mineralocorticoids—fludrocortisone 0.1 mg/day may be needed in some patients
- Treat infection, as this is a very common precipitating factor.

Section

7

Shock

Chapter

53

Hypovolemic Shock

- Shock is the clinical condition of organ dysfunction resulting from an imbalance between cellular oxygen supply and demand.
- Hypovolemic shock: reduction in cardiac output due to reduced preload secondary to reduced intravascular volume.

Causes

- Gastrointestinal—vomiting and diarrhea
- Renal—diuretic induced, osmotic diuresis, salt-wasting nephropathies, etc.
- Skin—excessive sweating, burns and erythroderma
- Third space sequestration—secondary to pancreatitis, acute febrile illnesses, intestinal obstruction, sepsis, fractures and crush injury
- Bleeding—internal/external—upper/lower GI bleeding, menorrhagia, trauma and ruptured aortic aneurysm
- Others—diabetic ketoacidosis, diabetes insipidus, etc.

Symptoms

- Secondary to hypovolemia
  - Lassitude, easy fatigability, thirst and muscle cramps
  - Postural giddiness
  - Decreased urine output
  - Lethargy, confusion and altered sensorium
- History pertaining to the cause of hypovolemia is to be elicited

Signs

- Dry tongue and sunken eyes
- Decreased skin turgor (not reliable, especially in elderly)
- Dry skin and axilla,cramps
- Tachycardia >100/min, precedes fall in BP
- Postural hypotension—>20/10 mm of Hg drop in systolic and diastolic >10% of blood volume loss.
- Supine hypotension <90 mm of Hg systolic (if >20% of blood volume is lost)
- Oliguria <0.5 mL/kg/hr
- Altered sensorium—if dehydration is severe

Investigations

- Elevated urea and creatinine, elevated BUN: Creatinine ratio
- Electrolytes—hypo-/hypernatremia, hypo-/hyperkalemia
- ABG—to look for metabolic acidosis/alkalosis
- Hb, hematocrit may be high due to dehydration
- Low urine sodium (in non-renal causes)
- USG—to look for IVC collapsibility
- Elevated lactate—for tissue perfusion

Management

Resuscitation

Fluid replacement—mainstay of treatment

- Place large bore canula for fast fluid replacement
- Crystalloids are preferred—NS/RL-1-2L bolus, followed by maintenance fluid based on fluid status
- Correct electrolytes, and acid–base disorders
- Blood transfusion for blood loss causing hypovolemia
  - Identify and treat cause of hypovolemia

Chapter 54

Septic Shock

Sepsis—a life threatening organ(s) dysfunction caused by a dysregulated host response to infection.

Septic shock—it is a subset of sepsis with hypotension with increased mortality risk. It can also be defined as:

A. Suspected infection (bacterial, viral, fungal and protozoal)

B. Vasopressor therapy required to maintain mean arterial pressure (MAP) >65 mmHg

C. Serum lactate >18 mg/dL despite adequate fluid resuscitation.

(MAP: Diastolic BP + $^1/_3$ pulse pressure)

Clinical Features

Symptoms

- Fever
- Symptoms specific to the source of the infection, e.g. cough, sputum, pain abdomen, urinary complaints and cellulitis
- Altered sensorium
- Oliguria

Signs

- Tachycardia (>90 bpm)
- Tachypnea (>20 respiratory rate)
- Hypotension (SBP <90 mmHg, MAP <65 mm)
- Hypoxia
- Warm peripheries initially. Later cold and clammy as the severe shock sets in.
- Obtundation and altered sensorium
- Other systemic examination based on the source of the infection and the pattern of organ dysfunction

q SOFA score (quick SOFA score)

It is an easy tool for quick recognition of sepsis in hospital or emergency triage. It ranges from 0 to 3 points and includes:

- Systolic hypotension (SBP <100 mmHg) — 1 point
- Tachypnea (respiratory rate >22 breaths/min) — 1 point

- Altered mentation — 1 point

A qSOFA score >2 points has a predictive value of sepsis. This score has poor specificity,and can overdiagnose sepsis.

Sequential Organ Failure Assessment score (SOFA score)

It is calculated within 24 hours of admission to an ICU. Useful for prognosis.

SOFA score	0	1	2	3	4
Respiration PaO_2/FiO_2 (mmHg) (kPa)	>400 >5.3	301–400 (4.1–5.3)	201–300 (2.8–4.0)	101–200 (1.4–2.7)	≤100 ≤1.3
Coagulation Platelets ($x10^3/mm^3$)	>150	101–150	51–100	21–50	≤20
Liver bilirubin (mg/dL) (µmol/L)	<1.2 <20	1.2–1.9 (20–32)	2.0–5.9 (33–101)	6.0–11.9 (102–204)	≥12.4 ≥204
Cardiovascular Hypotension	No hypotension	MAP <70 mmHg	Dopamine ≤5 or dobutamine (any dose)*	Dopamine >5	Dopamine >15
Central nervous system Glasgow Corma Score	15	13–14	10–12	6–9	<6
Renal Creatinine (mg/dL) (µmol/L) or urine output	<1.2 (<110)	1.2–1.9 (100–170)	2.0–3.4 (171–299)	3.5–4.9 (300–440) <500 mL/day	>5.0 >440 <200 mL/day

*Adrenergic a agents administered for at least 1 hour (does given are in µg/kg/min)

An admission SOFA score of >2, suggests prolonged hospital stay and bad prognosis.

Investigations

- CBC—leukocytosis or leukopenia
- Peripheral smear with neutrophils having toxic granules and immature forms (e.g. bands). It can also show evidence of schistocytes in case of DIC
- Thrombocytopenia
- Hyperglycemia or hypoglycemia
- Increased CRP levels (more than 2 standard deviations of the normal)
- Serum procalcitonin levels—maybe high in bacterial sepsis.
- RFT—high in sepsis induced AKI
- LFTS—high bilirubin/elevated liver enzymes as part of multiorgan dysfunction.
- Elevated lactate levels—usually >18 mg/dL
- ABG—high anion gap metabolic acidosis because of high serum lactate levels. It can also show hypoxia with reduced P/F ratio if ARDS is present.
- Microbiology—blood cultures and other site specific cultures must be sent as well, e.g. in case of pneumonia—respiratory cultures such as sputum, endotracheal or BAL cultures. Urine C/S in UTI.

- Chest X-ray for ARDS
- Imaging: USG/CT scan for pyelonephritis or abscesses
- ECG and ECHO—for sepsis induced myocarditis and for guiding fluid resuscitation based on cardiac status.

Immediate Management

This basically involves stabilizing patient, A – airway/B – breathing/C – circulation

- Securing the airway and treating hypoxia:
  - Intubation if the patient is hypoxic, or in respiratory fatigue/metabolic acidosis/altered sensorium.
- Adequate IV access:
  - Requires a central venous catheter preferably, for administration of IV fluids, inotropes especially.

Initial Resuscitation

Empirical antibiotics

- IV antibiotics should be initiated within 1 hour of recognition of sepsis after collecting the appropriate cultures. These are empirical, and must be relooked at when cultures become available.
- The choice of antibiotics depends on the source of infection, the most common microbes of that area and the hospital's antibiotic policy.
- **Broad-spectrum antibiotics**
  - Inj piperacillin tazobactam 4.5 g IV q8 h infused over 1–3 hours, or
  - Inj cefepime 2 g IV q8 h to q12 h.
  - Inj meropenem 1 gm IV 8th hourly given as an infusion over 3 hours.
  - If suspecting Gram-positive infections especially MRSA/Enterococcus:
    - Inj vancomycin 25 to 30 mg/kg IV loading dose followed by 15–20 mg/kg IV q8 h to q12 h or Inj teicoplanin 6–8 mg/kg IV q12 h for 3 doses followed by 6 mg/kg IV q24 h).
- Important:
  - Modify doses according to GFR, for renal failure
  - Change to appropriate antibiotics according to culture and sensitivity, and de escalate when necessary.
- **Fluid therapy:**
  - IV fluids at 30 mL/kg is to be given in the first three hours. (Either 0.9 % normal saline or ringer lactate).
  - Reduce in patients with fluid overload state, poor cardiac status or ARDS.
  - Resuscitation should continue until MAP of >65 mm Hg is reached.
  - For known hypertensives, a MAP of up to 75–85 mm of Hg can be targeted.

Inotropes

These should be initiated if target MAP is not reached with fluid resuscitation.

Norepinephrine first choice

- Dose: 0.1 to 3 μg/kg/min.
- Dilution: If taken as 8 mg in 42 mL normal saline, it can be started at 2 mL/hr (0.1 μg/kg/min) and can increased to 22 mL/hr (1 μg/kg/min).
- Doses higher than this is not usually given as it can causes gangrene and tachycardia.

Vasopressin is the next choice

- Dose: 0.03 units/minute
- Dilution: 40 units in 39 mL normal saline. It can be started at 1.2 mL/hr (0.02 units/minute) and increased to 2.4 mL/hr (0.04 units/minute).

Adrenaline can be started

- Dose: 0.01 to 0.7 μg/kg/min
- Dilution: 9 mL in 41 mL normal saline which can be started at 2 mL/hr (0.1 μg/kg/min) it can be increased to 22 mL/hr
- Avoid in severe lactic acidosis, as adrenaline causes an increase in lactate.

MONITORING OF ADEQUACY OF CIRCULATION

- If available, dynamic and static variables should be used to assess fluid responsiveness. Monitor:
  - Hourly urine output—more than 0.5 ml/kg/hr minimum.
  - IVC measurement for collapsibility
  - Serial lactate levels
  - Watch for clinical signs of fluid overload including raised JVP, basal crepitation with hypoxia.
- If the hypotension does not resolve with adequate fluid resuscitation and vasopressors, IV hydrocortisone 50 mg IV 6th hourly can be tried till MAP improves.

Supportive therapy

- Source control –

  Identifying the source of infection and controlling it by medical (IV antibiotics) or surgical (e.g. incision and drainage) should be attempted as soon as possible.
- Mechanical ventilation—ARDS for management (refer to Chapter 29: ARDS).
- Glucose control –
- Blood glucose should be monitored frequently and kept in the range of 110 to 180 mg/dL. Insulin should be initiated if more than 2 readings of blood glucose is >180 mg/dL.

Note

  - In patients with refractory hypotension, to check arterial blood glucose rather than peripheral blood glucose which might not be accurate.
  - Renal replacement therapy—for AKI with definitive indications of dialysis.
- Blood transfusion or platelets or FFP as needed.
- Nutrition—early enteral nutrition should be initiated if tolerated by the patient. Small balanced feeds should be initiated first which can then be increased based on tolerance.

The mnemonic **FAST HUGS BID** can be used for daily monitoring for all patients requiring ICU care. It provides an easy, quick way to monitor to a critically ill patient in an ICU setting.

F	Feeding
A	Analgesia
S	Sedation
T	Thromboprophylaxis
H	Head end elevation
U	Ulcer prophylaxis
G	Glycemic control
S	Spontaneous breathing trial, SpO_2
B	Bowel, bladder and bedsores
I	In dwelling catheters, intake/output
D	De-escalation of antibiotics

Chapter

55

Anaphylaxis

Anaphylaxis is a rapidly developing life-threatening multisystem syndrome caused by sudden release of mast cell mediators into systemic circulation after exposure to an allergen.

Diagnostic Criteria

Acute onset of illness (mins to hours) involving skin, mucosal tissue and at least one of the following:

A. Involvement of skin and mucosal tissues (generalised urticaria, hives, angioedema, flushing)
B. Respiratory compromise (stridor, wheeze, dyspnea, cyanosis)
C. Hypotension
D. Persistent gastrointestinal symptoms (abdominal pain, vomiting)

Clinical Assessment

- History of exposure to drugs/food (fish, egg, milk products-common)/insect bite/stings
- Check vitals: Low saturation/tachycardia/BP—hypotension/RR increased with dyspnea
- Evidence of allergy: Urticaria/angioedema/wheezing/stridor
- RS: For wheezing

Management

Remove source of anaphylaxis: Stop offending drug infusion. Remove stinger as in bites.

AIRWAY AND BREATHING

- Assess the patient for glottic/periglottic swelling by asking the patient to speak his/her name and look for edema of the lips, tongue and oropharynx.
- Supplemental oxygen: Using a non-rebreathing mask to maintain saturation
- If the patient has stridor or respiratory arrest intubation is required immediately.
- Prepare for an early intubation if there is significant edema of oropharyngeal tissue or glottic/periglottic swelling (voice alteration) as they can progress rapidly to respiratory arrest.
- Emergency cricothyroidotomy may be required if upper airway edema is severe.

Note

Intubation in the setting of upper airway edema may be difficult and hence should be attempted by an experienced clinician. If available an anesthesiologist/emergency team/otolaryngologist should be kept in the loop during accessing an airway for these patients.

CIRCULATION

- Immediately obtain two large-bore intravenous lines to administer fluids and medications.
- Place the patient in supine position and elevate the lower limbs
- In normotensive patients administer isotonic saline at a rate of 125 mL/hr to maintain venous access.
- Large volume fluid resuscitation is required in patients with hypotension, or incomplete response to epinephrine. 1–2 litres of normal saline should be administered as a bolus. May need up to 5–7 litres.

PHARMACOLOGICAL MANAGEMENT

1. EPINEPHRINE

The first and most important treatment for anaphylaxis

- Epinephrine: 1 mg/mL preparation may also be labelled as 1:1000
- Give epinephrine 0.3–0.5 mg intramuscularly, usually in the lateral mid thigh. Should be repeated every 5–15 minutes up to 3 doses till clinical improvement occurs
- If patients are not responding (up to 3 doses) prepare intravenous infusion of epinephrine.

Epinephrine Infusion

- Prepare a 4 μg/mL solution by adding 10 mL of 0.1 mg/mL epinephrine to 250 mL of normal saline.
- The resultant solution will deliver 1 μg/min of epinephrine in 15 mL/hr of infusion.
- Infusion rates: Start the infusion at 0.1 μg/kg/min and increase it by 0.05 μg/kg/min every 2–3 min till blood pressure improves.

Bolus IV Epinephrine

- If infusion is not readily available, push 0.05 to 0.1 mg of epinephrine over 1–3 minutes.
- Up to 2 doses can be repeated.

Local Administration of Epinephrine

- If clear bite mark, as in bee sting, or site of allergen is identified, epinephrine can be administered 0.1 mL locally.
- Tie a tourniquet above the bite mark, to slow down absorption.
- Keep patient in supine position before giving epinephrine to prevent decrease in venous return to heart (empty heart syndrome).

2. GLUCAGON

- Patients in anaphylaxis, taking beta-blockers may be refractory to epinephrine and hence glucagon should be administered.
- It is given as 1 mg slow IV bolus followed by infusion of 1 mg/hour to provide inotropic support.

Bronchodilators

- Inhaled bronchodilators with salbutamol can be used via nebulisation, if wheezing persists.
- Dose of 2.5 mg to 5 mg and repeated as necessary.

ADJUNCTIVE AGENTS

1. H_1 antihistamines
- Intravenous cetirizine 10 mg IV over 1–2 minutes.
- Intravenous diphenhydramine 25–50 mg over 5 minutes, which can be repeated every 4–6 hours to a maximum of 400 mg/day.
- H_2 antihistamines
- Ranitidine may be administered intravenously as 50 mg in 20 mL 5% dextrose given over 5 mins.

2. Glucocorticoids
- Maybe helpful to prevent the biphasic reactions that can occur in some patients.
- Acts after several hours.
- Intravenous hydrocortisone 100 mg IV 8th hourly for 1–2 days.
- Oral prednisolone can be continued for a few days at 1–2 mg/kg/day till the allergic reaction subsides.

Note

Steroids act late and should not be considered for emergency treatment in anaphylaxis. It can be considered in severe cases requiring hospitalisation, or in patients with asthma having bronchospasm in which symptoms have not subsided with other therapy.

Prevention

- Patient education regarding cause of allergy
- Wearing a bracelet to indicate risk of a particular drug/food, the patient is allergic to.

Section

8

Infections

Chapter

56

Severe Malaria

Caused by falciparum malaria and very rarely by vivax malaria. It should be suspected in individuals from endemic area or have travelled from high prevalence area.

Patients present with fever, anemia, hemolytic jaundice and mild firm splenomegaly.

Diagnosis of Severe Malaria

- It is associated with high parasitemia and major organ dysfunction
- WHO criteria for severe malaria:

Symptoms	Sign/Lab Investigations
Impaired consciousness	GCS <11 in adults, or Blantyre < 3 in children
Prostration	Generalized weakness
Multiple convulsions	More than 2 episodes in 24 h
Metabolic acidosis	HCO_3 <15 mmol/L, lactate >5 mmol/L
Hypoglycemia	RBS <40 mg/dL
Severe anemia	Hb <5 g/dL
Renal impairment	Creat >3 mg/dL, Urea >20 mg/dL
Jaundice	Total bilirubin >3 mg/dL
Pulmonary edema	Tachypnea, crepitations, CXR findings
Significant bleeding	Recurrent or prolonged mucosal or internal bleeding
Hyperparasitemia	*P. falciparum* >10%
Shock	Hypotension with SBP <90 mmHg

Investigations

Specific

- Malarial parasite by QBC technique
- Malaria antigen based tests (Falcivax)
- Peripheral smear—thick and thin smears. Repeat smear needed after 12–24 hours, if clinical suspicion is high
- Parasite Index*—percentage of RBC infested with parasite
  - 2–10%—indicates very severe infection.

**Parasite index and severity need not match*

Organ Dysfunction

- CBP—Hb (anemia), PCV, platelet count (low), TLC, DLC, ESR, repeat Hb, PCV 12th hourly)
- LFT (high bilirubin, mild to moderate rise in enzymes)
- RFT (urea, creatinine raised), electrolytes
- RBS—hypoglycemia due to parasite, hepatic dysfunction and renal failure (repeat 4th hourly)
- ABG for hypoxia and metabolic acidosis

Treatment

Specific: to be started as early as possible for better prognosis.

Artemisinin

Artemisinin derivatives (artesunate, artemether) preferred over quinine (AQUAMAT and SEQUAMAT study)

- Artesunate: 2.4 mg/kg IV at 0 hours, 12, 24 hours, and then once a day till patient can take orally.
- Artemether: 3.2 mg/kg on day one, 1.6 mg/kg daily after that, till the patient can take orally.
- IM/per rectal can be given if IV access not available
- No renal or hepatic dose adjustment needed

Quinine (as alternative second choice)

- Loading dose – 20 mg/kg in 5% dextrose over 4 hours
- Maintenance dose –
  - 10 mg/kg in 5% dextrose infusion over 4 hours q8 h, till patient is stable and fit for oral tablets. (Renal failure—50% of dose from day 3 onwards.)
  - If parenteral quinine therapy needs to be continued beyond 48 hours, dose should be reduced to 7 mg/kg 8 hourly.

Oral dose—10 mg/kg q8 h, total 7 days

Side effects: QT prolongation and hypoglycemia. Monitor with ECGs and RBS.

Note

If patients cannot take orally after 24 hours, doxycycline/clindamycin must be added to artesunate, especially in India.

Follow up oral drugs: Artemisinin combination therapy (ACT)

Once the patient can take orally:

For patients who were given artesunate

- Artesunate 4 mg/kg daily for 3 days plus sulphadoxine 25 mg/kg and pyrimethamine (1.25 mg/kg) on day 1) on day 1 **(ACT+AS)**
- For north eastern states: **ACT+AL**
- Artemether + lumefantrine (1.5 mg/9 mg/kg bid for 3 days)

For patients, who received quinine

- Quinine (10 mg/kg) plus doxycycline 100 mg bd for 7 days.
- In case of doxycycline is contraindicated (as in pregnancy and in children), clindamycin (450 mg tid) can be given.

On the second day of treatment, single dose of tab primaquine 0.25 mg/kg to eliminate gametocytes.

SYMPTOMATIC AND SUPPORTIVE CARE

- Close monitoring and ICU care
- Continuous vital sign monitoring—pulse, BP, temp, RR and SaO_2
- Secure IV lines—IV fluids, anti-pyretic,
- Oxygen, ventilator support and general care of a critically ill patient
- Care of unconscious patient

Cerebral malaria: Mortality 15–20% even with treatment

- Features: Unconsciousness, convulsions, no focal deficits
- Anti-cerebral edema measures—mannitol not useful. Use hypertonic saline 3% and hyperventilation.
- Anticonvulsants if there are convulsions. Not prophylactic.

Acute kidney injury

- Multifactorial; shock/hemoglobinuria
- Maintain fluid and electrolyte balance
- Hemodialysis if required
- Renal dose adjustment only required for quinine

Hypoglycemia

- Due to parasite, liver dysfunction and renal failure
- <40 mg/dL is dangerous
- 50 mL of IV 50% dextrose stat followed by 10% dextrose drip needed especially when quinine is being used.

Lactic acidosis (metabolic acidosis)

- Due to sepsis/hepatic and renal dysfunction/hypotension/RBC sequestration in small blood vessels
- Treat cause

Respiratory complications: ARDS/pulmonary edema

- ARDS due to cytokine storm. Can sometimes occur after malaria is treated
- Pulmonary edema due to cardiac dysfunction secondary to malaria and anemia
- Do not overhydrate
- Ventilate with low tidal volume, high PEEP

Secondary bacterial pneumonia

- Watch for secondary infection and treat with broad-spectrum antibiotics on an emergency basis.

Anemia

- Packed RBC transfusion if Hb is less than 7 gm %.

Thrombocytopenia

- Platelet transfusion if below 10,000 cells/cmm or less than 20,000 cells/cmm with significant bleeding.

Fluid management

- Patients can be in shock or pulmonary edema.
- Fluids must be managed on case to case basis.
- Watch for pulmonary edema.
- Support with inotropes if there is hypotension.

Exchange transfusion—not useful.

Malaria in pregnancy: Use artesunate/quinine as above. Clindamycin can be given. Doxycycline contraindicated.

Severe vivax malaria

Treat as per the falciparum malaria guidelines except for primaquine which is given at 30 mg/day for a total of 14 days.

Chapter

57

Leptospirosis

Caused by *Leptospira* species (especially *L. interrogans*)—a spirochete

- It is a zoonotic infection, caused by exposure to water/soil contaminated with animal (especially rodent) urine or tissue.

Common in farmers, field workers, people who handle animals.

Clinical Features

- *General:* Fever with chills, maculopapular rash, severe myalgia, conjunctival suffusion/hemorrhage, headache.
- *Organ dysfunction:* Jaundice, oliguria, renal failure, bleeding diathesis, aseptic meningitis, pancreatitis, respiratory distress and hypotension.
- *Biphasic disease*
  - Bacteremic phase—2–9 days.
  - Immune phase—recurrence of fever.

Investigations

General

- CBP—neutrophilic leukocytosis with thrombocytopenia
- RFT—renal failure. Can be significant
- LFT—raised bilirubin (marked) and transaminitis (mild to moderate <200). Amylase/lipase rise in some patients.
- Urine examination—proteinuria, granular casts in urine, microscopic hematuria, pyuria
- Elevated creatinine kinase
- Elevated amylase and lipase
- Chest X-ray—for ARDS/pulmonary alveolar hemorrhage
- ABG—type-1 respiratory failure
- ECG—myocarditis
- PT-INR and aPTT

Specific test in leptospirosis

Test	Sensitivity (%)	Specificity (%)	Time of maximum positivity
Microscopic agglutination test (MAT)—acute setting	55.3	95.7	7-10 days, Requires paired sample for best results
MAT—paired sample	Considered as gold standard/reference for comparison; Not commonly available		
Dark ground microscopy	Lesser sensitivity and operator dependent		Within 10 days
PCR—urine and blood for organism	50–60	80–100	Becomes positive within first 5 days
IgM ELISA	86	84.5	After 5–7 days

*MAT single value >1:800 represents recent or recurrent infection
* MAT paired—fourfold rise in titres between acute and convalescent serum is diagnostic

Treatment

1. **Antibiotics**—any one of the following

- Parenteral

Class	Drug	Dosage and frequency
Beta-lactams—first line	Crystalline penicillin	15–20 lakh units IV q6 h
	Ampicillin	1g IV q6 h
Cephalosporins	Ceftriaxone	2 g IV q24 h
	Cefotaxime	1g IV q8 h
Tetracyclines	Doxycycline	100 mg IV q12H
Macrolides	Azithromycin	500 mg IV od

Duration of treatment: 7 days

- Oral (for mild and OPD cases only)
  - Doxycycline 100 mg bd (for 7 days)
  - Azithromycin 500 mg od (for 3 days)
  - Amoxicillin 500 mg tid

In pregnancy—to avoid tetracyclines; prefer azithromycin and beta lactams

2. **Supportive**

- IV fluids—based on fluid status
- Cardiac and hemodynamic monitoring and support
- Management of renal failure—including hemodialysis if required
- Fresh frozen plasma/platelet transfusion—in case of bleeding manifestations.
- Respiratory support—oxygen/mechanical ventilation, if hypoxic/in ARDS

Role of steroids:

IV corticosteroids—for severe cases, especially with pulmonary hemorrhage

- IV methylprednisolone 1g od for 3 days, followed by tapering
- Controversial role, may benefit, but may also increase risk of nosocomial infections

Mortality and Prognosis

- Usually, with prompt initiation of appropriate antibiotics and supportive treatment, patients recover to normal functional status.
- Mortality of around 5% in hospitalised patients.

Chapter

58

Scrub Typhus

- It is a mite borne infection.
- Gram-negative coccobacillus, *Orientia tsutsugamushi.*
- Organism is inoculated into the skin of the host by the vector-trombiculid mites (larvae—chiggers).
- Mites and chiggers are present mainly in scrubs
- It has specific geographical prevalence within India, i.e. Karnataka, Tamil Nadu, Jammu and Kashmir, Himachal Pradesh, Bihar, Maharashtra and Rajasthan.

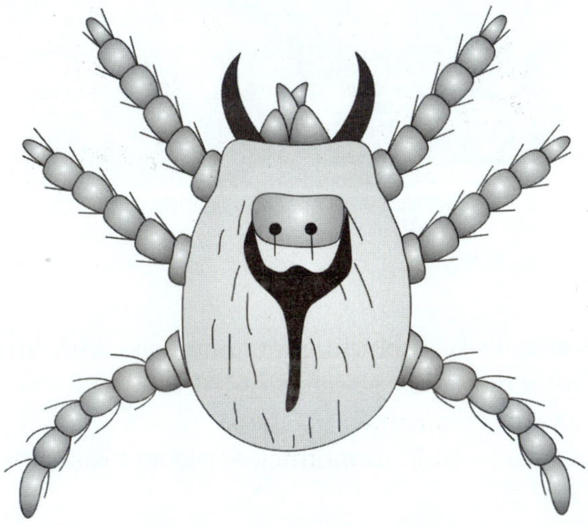

Fig. 58.1: Trombiculid mite

Clinical Features

- History of bite by mite—rarely reported by patients
- Address and occupational history—working in forests, near shrubs
- Fever with chills and rigors—7 to 10 days
- Headache
- Anorexia, nausea and vomiting
- Diffuse myalgia
- Rash—a diffuse non-pruritic, macular or maculopapular rash

- Eschar–
  - Painless papule appears at the site of the bite, with central necrosis, black crust and surrounding hyperemia
  - Found in the groin, lower abdomen or the perineal area—patient should be stripped and examined
  - Diagnostic of scrub typhus
- Local or generalized lymphadenopathy
- Hepatosplenomegaly
- Respiratory involvement in 10% cases with cough that can progress to ARDS
- Myocarditis and pulmonary edema
- Acute kidney injury
- In severe cases can cause meningitis or even encephalitis—with altered sensorium, seizures

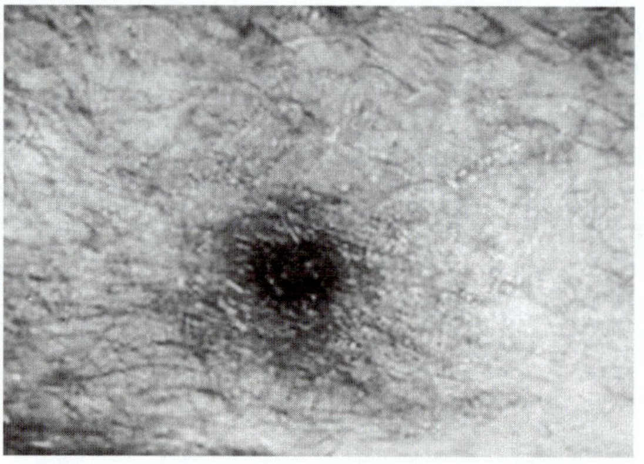

Fig. 58.2: Eschar seen in scrub typhus at the bite site

Investigations

General tests

- CBC—will show variable TC including leukocytosis, with thrombocytopenia
- LFT—elevated of liver enzymes, specifically ALP
- RFT—elevated urea and creatinine
- Cerebrospinal fluid (CSF)—mild mononuclear pleocytosis with normal glucose levels
- CXR—may show ARDS.

Specific Tests

	Test	When to test	Advantages/disadvantages
Weil felix	• Detects cross-reacting antibodies to proteus mirabilis OXK. • Shows ≥4 times rise in titre to proteus OXK • No reaction to proteus OX2 or OX19 • A single titer ≥1:160 is also diagnostic	• 5–10 days from onset • If done early, can be repeated	• Inexpensive test • Easy to perform • Quick results are available overnight • Lacks specificity and sensitivity

Contd.

(Contd.)

	Test	When to test	Advantages/disadvantages
Serology IgM IFA	• Detects specific antibodies – IgM type • Passive immunoassay • Fourfold increase in titres in paired samples drawn 14 days apart is diagnostic	• 5–7 days after onset • If done early, can be repeated	• Both sensitive and specific • IFA is the gold standard test
PCR	PCR amplification test Detects scrub antigen	• Done early in first week	• Most sensitive than specific test • Either from blood or eschar • Confirms the diagnosis

Treatment

Drug of choice

- Doxycycline 100 mg q12 h either oral or intravenously.
- Alternatives are tetracycline (500 mg q6 h) or azithromycin (500 mg PO, od, for 5 days),
- Duration: 7–14 days

Complications that require additional supportive care:

- ARDS—appropriate ventilation and oxygenation
- Myocarditis—may develop acute left heart failure, and hence fluid management becomes key here.
- Acute kidney injury—hydration and dialysis if required.

Clinical pearls

In clinical practice it is often difficult to differentiate leptospirosis from scrub typhus in endemic areas when the specific tests come negative

In scrub typhus, AST, ALT, ALP will rise disproportionately to bilirubin levels. Renal failure is not severe. The ALP may especially go up while on treatment, even when the patient is improving.

In leptospirosis, bilirubin is higher compared to AST/ALT rise, and kidney involvement can be severe.

Chapter

59

Dengue Fever

Caused by the dengue virus, a type of arbovirus, genus Flavivirus.

- Single stranded RNA virus, 4 serotypes
- Transmitted by the bite of the female aedes aegypti mosquito, more common in urban areas
- Breeds in domestic man-made water receptacles found in and around households, construction sites and factories
- Can present as:
  - Dengue fever
  - Dengue hemorrhagic fever
  - Dengue shock syndrome

Clinical Features: To be suspected in endemic areas

DF/DHF	Grade	Symptoms/signs	Laboratory findings
DF		Fever with two or more of following • Headache • Retro-orbital pain • Myalgia • Arthralgia	Leucopenia, thrombocytopenia
DHF	I	Above criteria for DF plus positive tourniquet test, evidence of plasma leakage	Thrombocytopenia: Platelet count less than 100,000/cu.mm. Hematocrit rise 20% or more
DHF	II	Above signs and symptoms plus some evidence of spontaneous bleeding in skin or other organs (black tarry stools, epistaxis, bleeding from gums, etc.) and abdominal pain	Thrombocytopenia platelet count less than 100,000/cumm Hematocrit rise 20% or more
DHF	III	Above signs and symptoms plus circulating failure (weak rapid pulse, pulse pressure ≤20 mm Hg or high diastolic pressure, hypotension with the presence of cold clammy skin and restlessness)	Thrombocytopenia: Platelet count less than 100,000/cumm Hematocrit rise more than 20%
DHF	IV	Profound shock with undetectable blood pressure or pulse Hematocrit rise more than 20%	Thrombocytopenia: Platelet count less than 100,000/cumm Hematocrit rise more than 20%

- Warning signs, (IV hydration, close monitoring required). To be looked for after the fever subsides, i.e. recovery phase in any dengue case.
  - Bleeding manifestations
  - Persistent high grade fever
  - Severe abdominal pain, persistent vomiting,
  - Dehydration
  - Impending circulatory failure or shock—tachycardia, postural hypotension, narrow pulse pressure, increased capillary refilling time > 3 secs
  - Neurological abnormalities—restlessness, seizures, altered sensorium

Investigations

1. CBC—usually thrombocytopenia can be profound, even <10,00 cells/cmm
2. Leukopenia is a feature < 3000 cells/cmm.
3. High Hb, and high hematocrit (>20%). Watch for rise in hematocrit which points to deterioration.
4. LFT can have increased AST and ALT (3–5 times) and hyperbilirubinemia (mild to moderate). Can be higher in DSS.
5. RFT-high in dengue shock
6. Chest X-ray and USG abdomen—for pleural effusion and ascites (during capillary leak)
7. Specific diagnostic tests:
   a. NS1 Ag-show positive result from day 1 to 5 (however can be positive for up to 12 days)
   b. Ig M antibody tests-use from day 5 onwards. IgG test will detect old infection
   c. Rapid diagnostic tests—detects IgG and IgM. It is rapid tests but exact sensitivity and specificity is not known.

Management

For dengue fever—supportive and symptomatic care:

- Bedrest
- Antipyretics for fever
- To avoid NSAIDs as it causes gastritis and platelet dysfunction
- Plenty of oral fluids and hydration—as shown in Flowcharts 59.1 and 59.2.
- Monitor for complications

Flowchart 59.1: Volume replacement flowchart for patients with DHF grades I and II

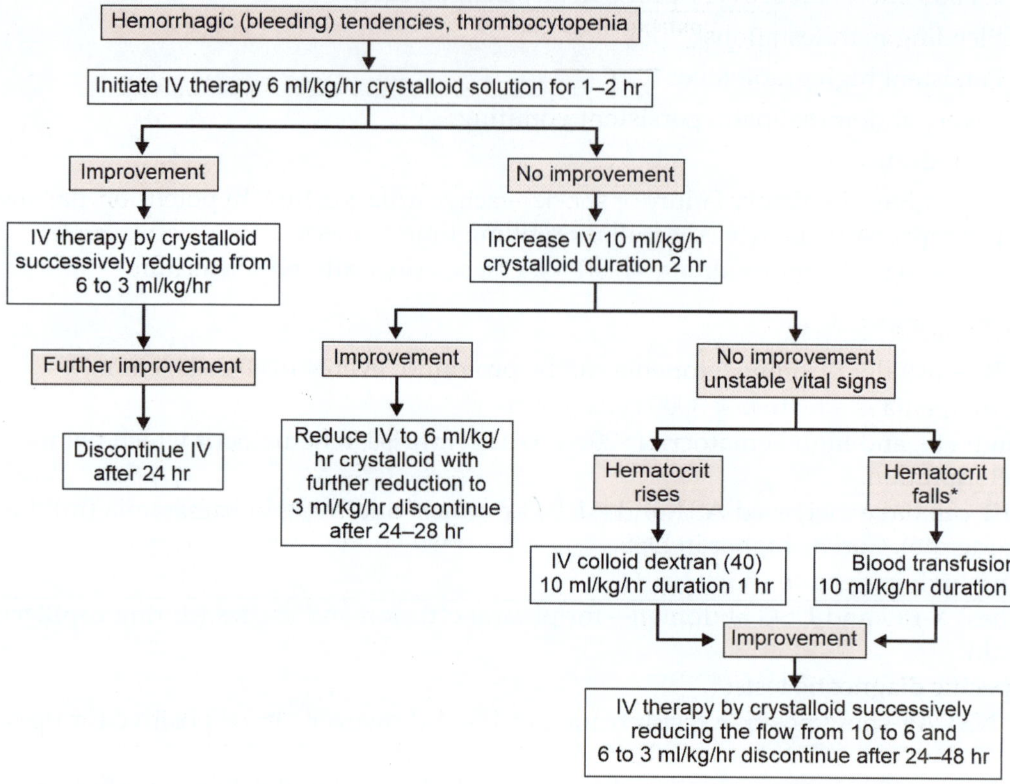

***Suspected internal hemorrhage**

Improvement : Hematocrit falls, pulse rate and blood pressure stable, urine output rises

No improvement : Hematocrit or pulse rate rises, pulse pressure falls below 20 mmHg, urine output falls

Unstable vital signs : Urine output falls, signs of shock

Supportive Therapy

- Hypotension usually develops after day 5 of the illness
- The above guidelines for fluid management—to be tailored based on cardiac status
- Indication for platelet transfusion
  - Significant bleeding manifestation at any platelet count
  - Prophylactic platelet transfusion, if <10,000 cells/mm^3

Flowchart 59.2: Volume replacement flowchart for patients with DHF grades III and IV

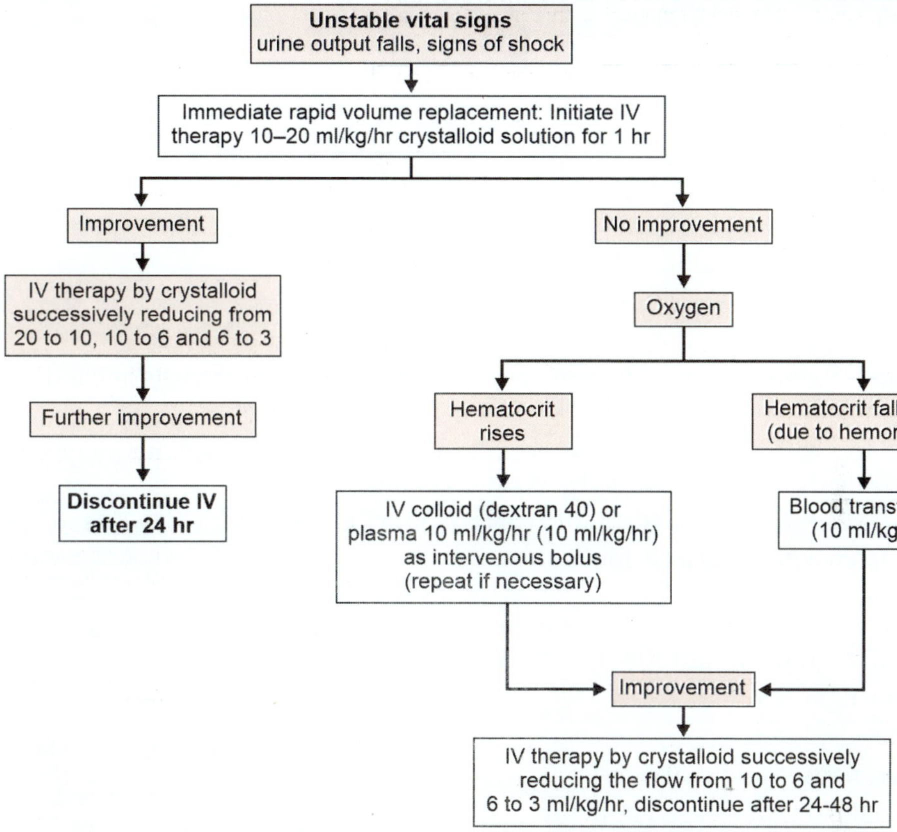

- Serial platelet and hematocrit determinations: Drop in platelets and rise in hematocrit are essential for early diagnosis of DHF
- Cases of DHF should be observed every hour for vital signs and urinary output

Recovery Phase

There is a recovery phase from dengue hemorrhagic fever—the capillary leak phase.

During this phase, the pleural fluid, etc. is reabsorbed, so we must tailor IV fluids to that. Otherwise patient may go into pulmonary edema.

Chapter

60

Kyasanur Forest Disease

- Organism—Kyasanur forest disease virus—an arthropod-borne virus of Flaviviridae family, transmitted by the hard tick—*Haemaphysalis spinigera*.
- Endemic to parts of Karnataka, especially in the Shivamogga, Chikmagalur and Uttara Kannada districts, along the Western Ghats.
- An outbreak of the disease is usually preceded by a sudden death of monkeys in the locality, from a hemorrhagic fever.

Symptoms and Signs

- Fever—high grade, intermittent, with chills
- Severe myalgia
- Headache
- Vomiting, nausea and diarrhea
- Abdominal pain/decreased appetite
- Bleeding manifestations—GI bleed, hematuria, gum bleed
- In severe cases—altered sensorium, seizures, myocarditis
- Occasional sinus bradycardia
- Hypotension—usually fluid responsive
- Bilateral cervical lymphadenopathy
- Rarely—erythematous rash

Second Phase

Around 2 – 4 weeks after recovery, may present with a second febrile phase, can have prominent neurological symptoms.

Complications

- Acute severe hepatitis
- Pancreatitis
- Myocarditis
- Encephalitis
- Severe bleeding

Investigations

General

- CBC—leukopenia (TC as low as 500/microL), with thrombocytopenia, with hemoconcentration; relative monocytosis
- LFT—marked transaminitis, low albumin and mild hyperbilirubinemia
- Creatinine phosphokinase—markedly elevated
- Hypocalcemia – corrected calcium as low as 5 mg/dL
- Amylase, lipase increased—in case of pancreatitis
- RFT—usually normal, may rarely have AKI
- Trop-T, NT-proBNP rise—in case of myocarditis
- Deranged coagulation profile—especially aPTT

Specific

- KFD: rT PCR—highly sensitive and specific
- Serology also available—IgM and IgG also available

In second phase—except for neutrophilic leukocytosis, other parameters are usually within normal limits.

Treatment: Supportive care only

- Hydration—IV fluids based on fluid status and oral fluids as tolerated
- Analgesics—for headache and myalgia
- Platelets and FFP transfusion—if bleeding manifestations (+)
- Vitamin-K injection (if PT/aPTT deranged)
- Empirical antibiotics maybe needed, if fever continues, neutrophil counts are very low, pending blood cultures.

Chapter

61

Resistant Enteric Fever

Caused by *salmonella enterica—S. typhi* and *S. paratyphi A* and *B*, which are Gram negative bacilli.

Caused by contact with food and water, contaminated with the bacteria—usually from another infected individual.

Symptoms and Signs

- Fever—high grade and usually continuous
- Headache
- Abdominal pain, nausea, vomiting, diarrhea
- Relative bradycardia
- Rose spots—faint salmon colored macules
- Just palpable soft spleen (in 2nd week of fever)
- Hepatomegaly

Complications

- Intestinal bleeding
- Intestinal perforation—Peyer's patch
- Myocarditis
- Typhoid encephalopathy
- Osteomyelitis (especially in individuals with sickle cell disease)
- Septic shock and ARDS

Investigations

General:

CBC—leukopenia with left shift. Eosinophil count close to zero. Platelets can be reduced.
LFT—transaminitis <5 times of normal

Specific

Blood culture:

- Positive in first week of illness (sensitivity—40–80%)
- Can be negative if already treated with antibiotics

Widal test:

- Positive from second week onwards
- Unreliable test

- Not reliable as high false positivity in endemic areas;
- False positive in active chronic hepatitis, rheumatoid arthritis, ulcerative colitis, past typhoid vaccination, malaria, dengue, disseminated TB, enterobacteriaceae
- False negative—early treatment with ampicillin or chloramphenicol, defect in antibody production
- Significant titre of 1:80 for O and 1:160 for H antigens.
- Titres higher than 1:640 more reliable
- 4-fold increase in titre is also significant (between first and second weeks)

*Stool and urine culture—third and fourth week (30-40% sensitive)

*Bone marrow aspirate culture—can be positive even with previous antibiotic treatment (sensitivity 55 – 90%)

Treatment

1. Antibiotics in Severe or Resistant cases

CLASS	Drug	Dosage and frequency
Cephalosporins for 10—14 days	Ceftriaxone (60—75 mg/kg/day)	**2 g IV q12 h**
	Cefotaxime	2g IV q8 h
Macrolides for 5–7 days	**Azithromycin (20 mg/kg–max 1 gm)**	**1g IV/PO STAT, followed by 500 mg/1 gm once daily**
Fluroquinolones (if sensitive) for 7–10 days	Ciprofloxacin	400 mg IV q12 h

Or, if the patient is stable and can tolerate orally,

- Cefixime 15–20 mg/kg/day PO twice daily
- Cefpodoxime 200–400 mg PO twice daily
- Ciprofloxacin 15 mg/kg or 750 mg PO twice daily
- Levofloxacin 500 mg PO once daily

Note

Preference—azithromycin > ceftriaxone > fluoroquinolone (Resistance common)

If it is a sensitive strain,

- Co-trimoxazole—double strength (160/800 mg)—around 50 to 60 mg/kg SMX in 3 divided doses for 10–14 days
- Chloramphenicol—50–100 mg/kg/day (maximum 3–6 g/day) in 4 divided doses for 2–3 weeks

For XDR strains, carbapenems can be given.

Duration of treatment is for 10–14 days (IV till patient is febrile/unstable; course can be completed orally when patient is better)

In suspected drug resistance or critically ill patients two drugs from different groups to be given.

2. General measures includes

- Bedrest
- Bland diet (avoid spicy food) and proper hydration

- Antipyretics
- Paracetamol 10 mg/kg/dose qid

Complications—management

- Intestinal bleeding—IV fluids and blood product transfusion
- Intestinal perforation—early surgical intervention carries a better prognosis compared to conservative management
- Typhoid state (delirium to coma)—antibiotic therapy and supportive care
- Typhoid shock—parenteral antibiotic therapy and management as septic shock
- Typhoid myocarditis—strict bedrest, fluid restriction and diuretics

Controversial role for high dose IV dexamethasone—for severe enteric fever with toxemia.

Chapter

62

Staphylococcal Bacteremia

Staphylococcus aureus is a leading cause of community-acquired and hospital-acquired bacteremia and infective endocarditis. Mortality rates **20 to 40%**, even higher with MRSA.

MRSA incidence ranges 2.3 to 69.1% in South and East Asia and the Western Pacific.

CLINICAL APPROACH

To find source: Potential portals of entry –

- Recent skin or soft tissue infection
- Intravascular, orthopedic and cardiac prosthesis/implantable devices.

For metastatic infection

For endocarditis: Look for stigmata of endocarditis
new regurgitant murmurs or heart failure

- **Bone or joint pain:** Vertebral osteomyelitis, discitis, epidural abscess
- **Abdominal pain:** Splenic infarction
- **Costovertebral angle tenderness:** Renal infarction or psoas abscess

Diagnostic Evaluation

Echocardiography for endocarditis. Transesophageal echo (TEE) is more sensitive than transthoracic echo (TTE) for identification of valvular vegetations.

Additional diagnostic imaging (especially vertebral column) based on history and clinical findings.

Treatment

- Prompt initiation of appropriate antimicrobial therapy
- Prompt and complete/effective source control (such as removal of implicated vascular catheters and/or drainage of purulent collections if present).

Empirical Therapy

Initially use vancomycin or daptomycin which have activity against methicillin-resistant *S. aureus* (MRSA).

If methicillin-sensitive *S. aureus* (MSSA), it is important to de-escalate to a beta-lactam agent, such as Co-amoxiclav, as vancomycin is considered inferior therapy for MSSA.

Treatment—MRSA Bacteremia

Recommended—vancomycin, teicoplanin or daptomycin

Vancomycin: Loading dose of 25–30 mg/kg followed by 15–20 mg/kg IV q8 h to q12 h Or

Teicoplanin: 8–12 mg/kg IV stat, same dose 8th hourly for day 1, followed by same dose od.

Daptomycin: 6–10 mg/kg/dose IV q24 h

For staph toxin: Add clindamycin/linezolid

Indication for Daptomycin

- Vancomycin MIC approaches the limit of the susceptible range (2 μg/mL)
- Poor initial clinical response (e.g., persistent bacteremia/clinical treatment failure)

Other Choices

- Ceftaroline: 600 mg IV q8 h
- Linezolid: 600 mg IV q12 h

Other regimens: In case of persistent and prolonged bacteremia, to avoid emergence of resistance.

- Daptomycin plus ceftaroline or other beta-lactams
- Vancomycin plus ceftaroline or other beta-lactams
- Daptomycin plus trimethoprim–sulfamethoxazole
- Ceftaroline plus trimethoprim–sulfamethoxazole

Note

- There is **no role** for quinupristin—dalfopristin, tigecycline, or fluoroquinolones for treatment of *S. aureus* bacteremia.
- Rifampicin is used in *Staph. bacteraemia* in the presence of prosthetic valve endocarditis or prosthetic joint infection with retained hardware.

In case of failure to clear bacteraemia within 48 hours after initiation of therapy:

- Clinical evaluation for occult focus of infection or persistent foci of infection (such as a deep-seated bone infection, abscess, retained prosthetic device, or endovascular source of infection) that may require drainage.
- Review of antibiotic susceptibility data

Treatment—MSSA bacteremia

Beta-lactam agent such as:

- Nafcillin (2 g IV q4 h), or
- Oxacillin (2 g IV q4 h), or
- Cefazolin (2 g IV q8 h), or
- Penicillin (4 million units IV q4 h) if sensitive

DURATION OF THERAPY

Once the diagnosis has been established and treatment has been initiated, follow up blood cultures should be repeated ideally every 24–48 h to document clearance of bacteremia

Uncomplicated *S. aureus* bacteremia may require—14 days of IV therapy **from the first negative blood culture**.

Complicated *S. aureus* bacteremia may require longer duration of IV depending on the clearance, 4–6 weeks.

Uncomplicated Infection

Must meet all the following:

- Exclusion of endocarditis by TEE
- No evidence of metastatic infection
- Definite and complete source control, i.e. removal of infected prostheses/indwelling catheter/drainage of abscess, etc.
- Blood cultures turn negative within 48–72 hours of instituting targeted antibiotic therapy
- Resolution of fever within 72 h of initiating effective therapy.
- Not immunosuppressed or neutropenic

Complicated Infection

Defined as: Patients with positive blood culture results who do not meet criteria for uncomplicated bacteremia.

Chapter

63

Tetanus

Caused by *Clostridium tetani*—Gram-positive, anaerobic, spore forming bacilli
History of wound contaminated by dust or soil.

Diagnosis

- History of injury
- 20–30% no entry wound seen
- Trismus, dysphagia and muscle stiffness
- Rigid abdomen, risus sardonicus, opisthotonos posture
- Hyperreflexia, autonomic dysfunction
- Episodes of generalized muscle spasms with cyanosis due to laryngeal spasm

Treatment of Tetanus

Admission in isolation ward or ICU—preferably in a dark, quiet room

Aims

1. Prevent further toxin release

a. Early and thorough wound debridement

b. Antibiotics for 7–10 days

- Inj metronidazole 500 mg IV q8 H/q6 h—preferred
- Inj crystalline penicillin 20–40 lakh units IV q4 h/q6 h

2. Neutralise unbound toxin

Inj human tetanus immunoglobulin (HTIG) 500 units IM-part around wound/ intrathecal injection—unproven benefit

3. Reduce effects of bound toxin

- Midazolam—preferred 0.2 mg/kg followed 0.05 to 2 mg/kg/hour
- If still uncontrolled—paralysis with
  - Vecuronium—0.08 to 0.1 mg/kg, then, IV infusion of 0.8 to 1.7 μg/kg/minute;
  - Cisatracurium—0.15 to 0.2 mg/kg f/b 0.01 mg/kg.
- Pancuronium is avoided as it may exacerbate autonomic symptoms
- Other drugs—dantrolene 1 mg/kg IV

  Baclofen—intrathecal 40–200 μg bolus f/b 20 μg per hr infusion

4. Autonomic instability

- Treated with morphine 0.5 to 1 mg/kg/hr
- Labetalol 0.25 1 mg/min or esmolol 500 μg/kg f/b 50 μg/kg/minute
- Magnesium sulphate (for muscle spasm as well as autonomic disturbance)
  - Loading dose 40 mg/kg over 30 mins,
  - Followed by infusion of 2 g per hour for patients >45 kg, or
    - 1.5 g per hour for patients ≤45 kg
    - Target plasma concentration of 2–4 mmol/L
  - Titrate with disappearance of patellar reflex

5. Supportive Care

- Hydration, nutrition and electrolyte management.
- ET intubation/tracheostomy and mechanical ventilation for hypoxia

Prognosis

- Case fatality is 40–50% in developing countries.
- Prognosis depends on effective supportive care and ICU facilities.
- Recovery takes 4–6 weeks.
- Patients must be given full primary immunization course following recovery

Tetanus Prophylaxis

Previous doses of tetanus toxoid	Clean and minor wound		All other wounds	
	TT vaccine	Immune globulin	TT vaccine	Immune globulin
<3 doses or unknown	Yes Give inj tetanus toxoid (TT) 0, 1, 6 months (Total 3 injections 0.5 cc IM)	No	Yes	Yes*
≥3 doses	Only if last dose given ≥10 years ago	No	Only if last dose given ≥5 years ago	No

*Injection human tetanus immunoglobulin 250 units IM at a different site than TT

Chapter

64

Acute Complicated UTI—Pyelonephritis

Clinical Features

- Fever with chills and rigors (always indicates involvement of upper urinary tract)
- Dysuria, lower abdominal pain, and loin pain
- Renal angle tenderness
- Features of MODS/septic shock—if severe

Predisposing Factors

- Diabetes (emphysematous pyelonephritis)
- Obstruction of urinary tract (BPH/stricture)/vesicourinary reflux)

Investigations

- CBP—TC increased. Neutrophilia
- CRP—increased
- Urine microscopy—for pus cells
- Urine culture and sensitivity—for organism
- Blood culture—for bacteremia
- Biochemistry: RFT/serum electrolytes—to assess renal dysfunction.
- Blood sugars for diabetes
- Procalcitonin—positive in bacteremia

INDICATIONS FOR IMAGING

USG

Look for kidney size/pyelonephritis/obstructive uropathy, renal abscess.

CT KUB

- Non-contrast CT—if creatinine is raised
- Contrast CT—if renal function is normal
- Defines obstructive uropathy/abscesses and kidney size better.

Organisms causing UTI

1. *E.coli*—commonest
2. Klebsiella

3. Proteus
4. Enterobacter
5. Pseudomonas
6. Enterococci
7. *Staphylococcus aureus*

Treatment in patients who have no MODS/septic shock

Inj ceftriaxone 2 gm IV od
Inj ciprofloxacin 400 mg IV bd
Inj gentamicin/netilmycin/3–5 mg/kg/day IV od/amikacin 15 mg/kg/day IV od

Treatment in patients who are seriously ill: Empirical therapy

- Cefeprazone sulbactum 1–3 gm IV q12 h, or
- Cefepime 1–2 gm q 12 h IV
- Ceftazidime 1 gm IV q8–12 h or
- Pipercillin tazobactum 4.5 gm IV 8th hourly
- Meropenem 1 gm IV 8th hourly
- Imipenem 500 mg IV every 6 hours, or
- Doripenem 500 mg IV every 8 hours

These have to be changed based on sensitivity reports, when they are available.

For resistant organisms (acinetobacter)

Colistin 9 million units IV stat, 3 million 12th hourly

For *Enterococcus faecalis*: Change catheter

Inj ampicillin 2 gm IV 6th hourly

For *Enterococcus faecium*/MRSA

Inj vancomycin 15–20 mg/kg loading dose, followed by 15 mg/kg IV 12th hourly

Vancomycin Resistant Enterococci

- Linezolid 600 mg IV bd
- Daptomycin 6 mg/kg IV infusion q24 h. For endocarditis, use 10 mg/kg.

Note

- Duration of treatment: 7–14 days
- Deescalate based on clinical findings, and biochemical recovery
- All antibiotics may have to be dose modified in renal failure, based on GFR.

Interventions

DJ stenting: Done if the patient has an obstruction in ureters causing hydroureteronephrosis, to relieve the block, and drain pus if collected in kidney. Needs to be removed after 1 month.

Percutaneous nephrostomy (PCN): For those who cannot undergo DJ stenting and need relief from obstruction of urinary tract

Milder UTI are treated with

- Ciprofloxacin 500 mg PO q12 h, or
- Cotrimoxazole DS PO q12 h

Recurrent UTI

- May need prophylaxis with CO-TDS—1 tab a day
- Nitrofurantoin—100 mg daily

Chapter

65

Lung Abscess

Formation of an abscess within lung parenchyma, with plenty of sputum.

Organisms Responsible

1. Anaerobes (bacteroides, fusobacterium, anaerobic and microaerophilic cocci and streptococci)
2. Gram-positive:
   - *Staphylococcus aureus*
   - *Streptococcus pneumoniae*
3. Gram-negative:
   - *Klebsiella pneumoniae*
   - *Pseudomonas aeruginosa*

Clinical Features

- High grade fever with chills and rigour—acute or subacute duration
- Plenty of purulent sputum/halitosis
- Hemoptysis
- History of aspiration,due to situations causing loss of consciousness: Seizure, anesthesia for surgery/stroke, etc.
- Clubbing +
- Auscultation-cavernous bronchial breathing and crepitations

Investigations

- CBP, peripheral smear
- Chest X-ray shows cavity with air fluid level
- CT chest for cavities
- Sputum cultures
- Blood cultures

Treatment in a Normal Host

Most of the cases are due to anaerobes and the patients will respond to

1. Inj cyrstalline penicillin 10 lakh units IV q6 h
   Or
2. Inj amoxyclav 1.2 gm IV q8 h
   Or
3. Clindamicin 600 mg IV q8 h

Treatment in a patient with a damaged lung, or

If the aspiration has occurred in the hospital

1. Inj piperacillin tazobactum 4.5 gm IV 8th hourly
   For MRSA and MSSA
   Refer to chapter on treatment of Staphylococcus infections

Duration of therapy:

Lung abscess 4–6 weeks
2 weeks of IV drugs + 4 weeks of oral therapy

If patient is stable/follow up therapy any of these can be chosen, depending on the organism grown in culture;

Amoxiclav 1 gm bd
Levofloxacin 500 od can be given
Clindamycin 600 mg tid

Supportive therapy:

- Chest physiotherapy
- Postural drainage
- Steam inhalation
- Mucolytics

Note

If the abscess does not communicate with the bronchus, the patient may continue to run high grade fever, and not bring out sputum. In such cases, a therapeutic bronchoscopy to establish communication with bronchus, may aid in drainage.

Chapter

66

Necrotising Fasciitis

Dangerous soft tissue infection of fascia, with secondary necrosis of underlying muscle and overlying subcutaneous tissues.

- Spreads very fast/high mortality
- Commonest risk factor: Diabetes

Etiology

- Monomicrobial—group A beta hemolytic Streptococcus
- Polymicrobial—mixed anaerobes and aerobes (Staphylococcus, *E. coli*, Proteus, Klebsiella, Pseudomonas, Bacteroids, etc.)
- Gas gangrene—most commonly due to Clostridium

Clinical Features

Predisposing factors:

- Diabetes mellitus
- Chronic liver disease
- Immunocompromised conditions

Presentation

- Fever—can be high grade
- Begins as small wound, but spreads very fast in involve whole limbs.
- Absence of gross redness, warmth maybe misleading regarding the severity of the illness.
- Pain severe and disproportionate to the findings on examiantion
- Crepitus

Blebs: Violaceous fluid filled blebs begin to appear on affected limb.

- This is the hallmark of the disease.
- It can spread very fast with lymphangitis and local lymph node involvement
- Gas formation maybe present

  Always remember to lift the limb and see for blebs, as it may form on that side, and easily missed.

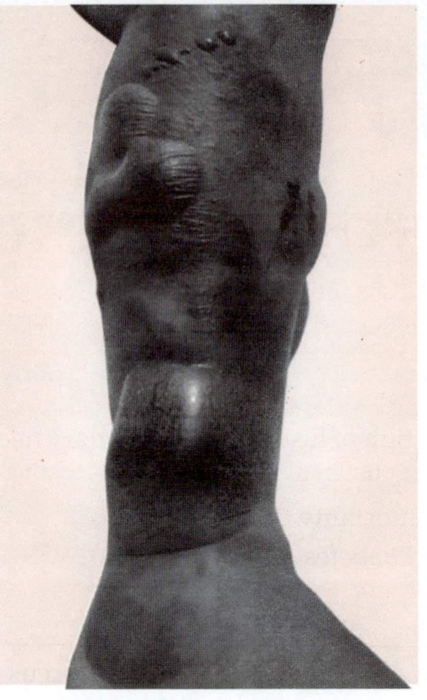

Complications

- Can progress to sepsis and septic shock.
- Compartment syndromes with necrosis of muscle and compression of arteries.

Investigations

- Leukocytosis and neutrophilia
- Increased CRP.
- Fasting blood sugars/postprandial sugars and HbA1c—for DM.
- Elevated CK and AST rise in muscle necrosis.
- RFT/LFT abnormal in case of sepsis rhabdomyolysis.
- Blood culture—may identify bacteremia.
- Pus culture—for organism
- X-ray or CT scan to show gas and abscess under the skin
- Biopsy of fascia to show necrosis—intraoperative

Treatment

Broad spectrum antibiotic to cover Gram-positive, Gram-negative and anaerobic organisms:

- Inj piperacillin tazobactam 4.5g IV q8 h infused over 1–3 hours, or
- Inj cefepime 2 g IV q8 h to q12 h, or
- Inj meropenem 1 gm IV 8th hourly given as an infusion over 3 hours.

If suspecting Gram-positive infections especially MRSA/Enterococcus: Any one of the following can be used in addition to above.

- Inj vancomycin 25 to 30 mg/kg IV loading dose followed by 15–20 mg/kg IV q8 h to q12 h, or
- Inj teicoplanin 6 mg/kg IV q12 h for 3 doses followed by 6 mg/kg IV q24 h), or
- Inj linezolid IV 600 mg IV 12th hourly for vancomycin resistant organisms.

Inj clindamycin 600–900 mg IV 8th hourly, can be added to above antibiotics, mainly to halt toxin production, if clinical picture fits toxic shock syndrome.

Hyperbaric oxygen has been tried with variable success

Surgery: This is a surgical emergency

- Debridement to remove all necrotic tissue is the most important aspect of management. This must be wide and extensive.
- This should be done early in the course of the illness.
- Can be lifesaving and limb-saving.
- Several debridements maybe needed for complete healing.

Supportive care

- Treatment of hyperglycemia with insulin
- Inotropes for septic shock
- Mechanical ventilation for ARDS

Prognosis

- Guarded
- Depends on host factors and virulence of organism.
- Early intervention is important to save life and limb.

Chapter

67

Febrile Neutropenia

It is more common in patients with malignancies but can also occur in other cases.
It is defined as:

- *Fever:* Oral temperature of >101°F (38.3°C) or a temperature of 100°F (38.0°C) sustained for > 1 hour period.

Definition

Neutropenia: An absolute neutrophil count <1500 cells/mm^3

- Severe neutropenia—<500 cells/mm^3 or anticipated decline in ANC to <500 cells/mm^3 in 48 hours
- Profound neutropenia—<100 cells/mm^3

Patients should be risk stratified into:

1. *Low risk:*
   - Expected duration of neutropenia is <7 days,
   - With no comorbid condition,
   - Stable renal and hepatic functions.
2. High risk:
   Expected to have a longer duration of neutropenia > 7 days
   - Hemodynamic instability
   - Renal and hepatic dysfunction
   - Systemic infections
   - Advanced age
   - Metastatic disease/acute leukemia or MDS during induction chemotherapy
   - Chronic lung disease/new pulmonary infiltrate or hypoxemia
   - Intravascular catheter infection

Management

Febrile neutropenia:

- Identify possible sources of infection
- Antibiotics should be started as soon as possible (within 2 hours in high risk patients).

Diagnosis

- History and physical examination:
  - Careful history to identify any clues to the source of infection.
  - Detailed examination for source including skin, vascular access catheter sites, to look for signs of inflammation.

Lab investigations

- CBP, LFT, RFT Na, K, Mg, Ca, P and alkaline phosphatase when needed
- A set of 2 blood cultures should be sent promptly (one from a peripheral vein and one if CLRBSI is suspected).
- If fever >48 hours, repeat blood cultures.
- Fungal infections like aspergillosis: Serum β-D-glucan and β-galactomannan
- Other cultures should be sent based on clinical suspicion. For example, in case of purulent discharge from the central venous catheter site, a swab should be sent for Gram stain, bacterial and fungal culture.
- Chest X-ray, X ray PNS, CT thorax for aspergillosis for neutropenia >1 week

Treatment

- Low risk patients: Oral antibiotics/IV antibiotics with close follow up.
- High risk patients: Admission mandatory, treat with IV antibiotics.

The empirical therapy should be based on local resistance pattern and cover both Gram-positive and Gram-negative bacteria.

Initiation of monotherapy with agent with broad spectrum including antipseudomonal coverage such as:

- inj cefepime (2 g IV q8 h),
- inj meropenem (1 g IV q8 h),
- Inj imipenem—cilastatin (500 mg – 1 gm IV q6 H)
- Inj piperacillin tazobactam (4.5 g IV q8 h)
- Aminoglycosides, fluoroquinolones, and/or vancomycin should be added as per the clinical findings.
- All these are better given as infusions over 3–4 hours to maintain minimum inhibitory concentration.

The antibiotics should then be changed based on the final culture and sensitivity report.

For urinary catheter related infection (Staphylococcus and Enterococcus)

- Vancomycin loading dose of 25 mg/kg, followed by (15 mg/kg–20 mg/kg per dose 12th or 8th hourly) or teicoplanin 6–8 mg/kg IV 12th hourly for 3 doses, followed by 6 mg/kg IV od can be added.

For suspected intra-abdominal infection:

In addition to broad-spectrum coverage mentioned above, anaerobic coverage should be added (neutropenic typhlitis). Inj metronidazole 500 mg tid IV.

Fever > 1 week

In case of persistent fever for more than 4 to 7 days in high-risk patients, antifungals can be started empirically.

For Candida grown in blood:

- If clinically stable: Inj fluconazole 800 mg IV loading dose, followed by 400 mg IV od
- If unstable:
  1. Liposomal amphotericin B 3–5 mg/kg IV daily
  2. Anidulafungin: 200 mg loading dose, then 100 mg intravenously (IV) daily
  3. Caspofungin: 70 mg loading dose, then 50 mg IV daily

4. Micafungin: 100 mg IV daily should be treated for *1 week after the last negative blood culture,* and until total counts improve.

For aspergillus

- CT scan of the thorax, and galactomannan needed for diagnosis
- Inj voriconazole
  - Initial: 6 mg/kg every 12 hours for 2 doses
  - Maintenance dose: 4 mg/kg every 12 hours
  - Treated for 12 weeks. Oral dose 200 mg bd

Catheter-related infections: 2 sets of cultures—one from peripheral line and one from central line

Central venous catheter should be removed for patients with catheter-related bloodstream infections caused by:

- Coagulase negative—*Staphylococcus aureus*
- *Staph. aureus*
- Enterococcus
- *Pseudomonas aeruginosa*, Klebsiella/*E.coli*
- *Candida* spp

Most infections need removal of the catheter. Treatment with appropriate drugs needed for 5–7 days after removal of catheter.

Prophylaxis

1. Antibiotic prophylaxis
   a. Fluoroquinolone prophylaxis: high-risk patients with expected durations of prolonged and profound neutropenia (ANC <100 cells/mm^3 for >7 days
   b. Levofloxacin (500 or 750 mg orally once daily) and ciprofloxacin (500 to 750 mg orally twice daily)
2. Fungal prophylaxis
   a. Patients with persistent or recurrent fever after 4–7 days of antibiotics and whose overall duration of neutropenia is expected to be >7 days
   b. Against Candida infection is recommended in:
      - Allogeneic hematopoietic stem cell transplant (HSCT) recipients, or
      - Those undergoing intensive remission-induction or salvage-induction chemotherapy for acute leukemia
      - Fluconazole 400 mg od
   c. Against invasive Aspergillus
      - Patients >13 years of age, undergoing intensive chemotherapy for acute myeloid leukemia (AML) or myelodysplastic syndrome (MDS)
      - *Tablet posaconazole*—loading dose 300 mg q12 h on day 1, followed by 300 mg od
3. Granulocyte—macrophage colony stimulating factors (Filgrastim)
   - Can be used in either prophylaxis or treatment.
   - It is considered only in high risk patients, e.g. in whom the anticipated risk of fever and neutropenia is ≥20%.
   - Dose: Filgrastim 5 microgm/kg/day
   - In case of treatment, it reduces the time to neutrophil recovery and duration of febrile neutropenia.

Section

9

Toxicology and Bites

Chapter

68

First Aid in Poisoning

Assessment of the Patient

- The level of consciousness
  - Agitation: Anticholinergic poisoning, central hallucinogens, drug withdrawal
  - Depression: Sedatives, hypnotics and ethanol poisoning
- Respiration and cyanosis
- Smell near the patient and gastric contents
- Pulse and blood pressure
- Presence of convulsions
- Size of the pupils
  - Small: Opiate, barbiturate and OP poisoning
  - Large: Cocaine abuse, atropine, tricyclic antidepressant poisoning
- Condition of the skin
- Any evidence of external injury
- Smell near the patient and gastric contents—important clue
- Circumoral staining or corrosion

- **Investigations**
  - RFT, serum electrolytes, serum osmolality, CK
  - ABG
  - RBS-hypoglycemia/hyperglycemia
  - LFT, PT—liver dysfunction, coagulopathy
  - Pseudocholinesterase for OP poisoning
  - Pregnancy testing
  - ECG—bradycardia, SVT, VT, QT prolongation
  - Imaging: X-ray, ultrasound, CT, MRI
  - Stomach contents, urine, blood for toxicology screening

Immediate Measures

Airway

- Maintenance of clear airway
- Oropharyngeal airway
- Endotracheal intubation

Breathing

- Supplemental oxygen
- Ventilatory support: If spontaneous ventilation is inadequate/hypoxia.
- Bronchodilators for bronchoconstriction

Maintenance of circulation:

- If the BP is low
  - Elevation of the foot end of the bed
  - Start IV fluids/inotropes
- If BP is high-start antihypertensives
- Treatment of cardiac arrest and arrhythmias (refer to the chapter on cardiopulmonary arrest).

TREATMENT OF POISONING

Removal of poison:

- Decontamination of the poison
- Remove contaminated clothes
- Wash the skin
- Irrigate the eyes with saline/water

Gastric Aspiration and Lavage

- It is useful especially within the first 4 hours after ingestion of the poison.
- Even later it should be tried, as it is the easiest method to remove the poison from the stomach.

Gastric Lavage

- Patient should be placed on their left side
- Lubricate the aspiration tube with glycerine
- Ensure that the tube is not misdirected into the larynx
- Pass up to 50 cm in adults (measured from the teeth)
- Aspirate the gastric contents completely
- 250–300 mL of warm saline or plain water at a time should be run and aspirated repeatedly till exit fluid is clear and odourless.

Contraindications are

- Corrosive poisoning
- Paraffin, kerosene, petrol, diesel and turpentine poisoning
- Unconscious patients without cuffed endotracheal tube in place
- Children (in whom emetics are preferred)

Emesis—Not used routinely

- Preferred method in children
- Should not be used in semiconscious or unconscious patients
- Syrup of ipecacuanha 15–30 mL orally
- This can be repeated once if there is no response

Activated charcoal as an adsorbent

- Dose 1 gram/kg (through RT) in divided doses
- Should be administered within 1–3 hours after ingestion of poison and it is not a substitute for adequate gastric lavage.

Whole-Bowel Irrigation

- Bowel preparation solution is administered at 2 L/h by gastric tube (children: 500 mL/h), until rectal effluent is clear or a total of 10–15 L have been passed
- **Indications**
  - Large ingestions of iron, lithium, or other drugs poorly adsorbed to activated charcoal.
  - Large ingestions of sustained—release or enteric-coated tablets containing valproic acid, theophylline, aspirin, verapamil, diltiazem.
  - Ingestion of foreign bodies or drug—filled packets or condoms.
- **Contraindications**
  - Ileus or intestinal obstruction.
  - Obtunded, comatose, or convulsing patient unless the airway is protected.

Supportive care

- Care of the unconscious patient (refer to chapter on approach to an unconscious patient)
- Treatment of convulsions (refer to the chapter on status epilepticus)
- Treatment of hypothermia
- Treatment of pyrexia
  - Few poisons themselves cause pyrexia
  - Look for the focus of infection, e.g. aspiration pneumonia

Specific Antidotes

- Available only for very few poisons.
- Refer to the table given as follows.

Poisons	Antidotes
Organophosphorus compounds	Atropine sulphate, pralidoxime chloride
Acetaminophen	N-acetylcysteine
Methemoglobinemia	Methylene blue
Ethylene glycol	Ethanol
Opioid	Naloxone hydrochloride
Carbon monoxide	Oxygen
Anticholinergics	Physostigmine

Indications for Hemodialysis

- Severe poisoning with methanol, ethanol, lithium, salicylates, phenobarbitone.
- Renal failure due to poisoning like copper sulphate.
- Hemoperfusion for paraquat poisoning

Summary of Toxidromes

Toxidrome	Mental status and pupils	Vital signs	Other manifestations	Examples of toxic agents
Sympathomimetic	Agitated pupils: Dilated	Hyperthermia Tachycardia Hypertension Tachypnea	Increased sweating Tremors, seizures Arrhythmias	Cocaine, amphetamines
Cholinergic	Confusion, coma, pupils: Small	Bradycardia Hypertension or hypotension Tachypnea or bradypnea	Salivation Lacrimation Urinary incontinence Diaphoresis Diarrhea Emesis	Organophosphate and carbamate insecticides
Anticholinergic	Agitated Hyperactive delirium Pupils: Dilated	Hyperthermia Tachycardia Hypertension Tachypnea	Flushing Dry skin and mucous membranes Decreased bowel sounds Urinary retention	Tricyclic antidepressant Atropine Anti-histamine Anti-spasmodic
Opioid	CNS depression, coma Pupils: Small	Bradypnea/ Apnea Hypothermia Bradycardia Hypotension	Pulmonary edema	Heroin, morphine, methadone, oxycodone, hydromorphone
Sedative-hypnotic	CNS depression, confusion, stupor, coma Pupils: Variable	Hypothermia Bradycardia Hypotension Apnea/ Bradypnea	Hyporeflexia Ataxia	Benzodiazepines Barbiturates Alcohols
Serotonin syndrome	Confusion, agitation, coma Pupils: Dilated	Hyperthermia Tachycardia Hypertension Tachypnea	Tremor Flushing Rigidity Diarrhea	MAOIs

Chapter

69

Organophosphorus (OP) Poisoning

Compounds: Chlorpyrifos, acetamide, dimethoate, ethyl and methyl parathion, quinalphos, diazinon, monocrotophos, etc.

Mechanism of Action

- Organophosphorus compounds bind to acetylcholinesterase (AChE) and render this enzyme non-functional. This leads to an abundance of acetylcholine.
- After a period of time the acetylcholinesterase—OP undergoes a conformational change, known as "aging," which makes the enzyme irreversibly resistant to reactivation by an oxime. Hence, early treatment is important.

Clinical Features

Cholinergic excess (muscarinic features)—*"DUMBBELLS"*

- **D**efecation
- **U**rination
- **M**iosis
- **B**ronchorrhea—pulmonary edema/**b**ronchospasm/**b**radycardia
- **E**mesis
- **L**acrimation
- **S**alivation/sweating

Nicotinic Symptoms

- Muscle fasciculations, cramps
- Muscle weakness, and paralysis

Neurological:

- Anxiety, confusion, delirium and hallucinations
- Seizures and coma

Respiratory complications: Respiratory failure

- Due to neuromuscular weakness due to nicotinic effect
- Depression of the CNS respiratory center
- Excessive respiratory secretions
- Bronchoconstriction

Intermediate syndrome:

- 10–40% of patients develop
- 24–96 hours after exposure.
- Neck flexion weakness, decreased deep tendon reflexes, cranial nerve abnormalities, proximal muscle weakness, and respiratory insufficiency
- May last 2–3 weeks and need ventilatory support.

Risk factors for intermediate syndrome:

- Exposure to a highly fat-soluble organophosphorus agent.
- Inadequate doses of oximes.

Cardiac

- Cardiac arrhythmias, including heart block and QTc prolongation
- 1/3rd patients may have myocardial ischemia, suggested by elevated troponin or changes in the ECG.

Investigations

- Toxic screen to assess gastric contents for OP
- CXR/ABG to assess respiratory status
- Serum pseudocholinesterase or RBC acetylcholinesterase
- Other routine biochemistry and hematology as baseline

Diagnosis

- History + clinical features suggestive of OP
- Characteristic petroleum or garlic-like odor, either on patient, or RT aspirate.
- Measurement of RBC acetylcholinesterase (RBC AChE) can be used to check the degree of toxicity.
- Serum cholinesterase (pseudocholinesterase) levels can be used if RBC AChE is unavailable
- Initial depressed level correlates with severity and prognosis.

Management: Decontamination—remove poison

- Complete removal of the patient's clothes and vigorous irrigation of the body and eyes
- Gastric lavage to remove OP.
- Activated charcoal 1 gram/kg every 4–6 hourly for 1 day to delay absorption
- Forced emesis is contraindicated in view of risk of aspiration.

Initial Resuscitation: Indications for Intubation and Ventilation

- Altered mental status
- Hypoxia/poor respiratory effort.
- Secretions/severe bronchoconstriction
- Succinylcholine should be avoided as it is metabolized by acetylcholinesterase leading to prolonged neuromuscular blockade.
- Based on ABG and CXR—intubate and ventilate
- Ventilation may be needed for weeks, especially if intermediate syndrome sets in.

Resuscitation

Bradycardia and hypotension: Fluid resuscitation.

Supportive Therapy

- IV fluids for nutrition and hydration, as patients cannot be fed through RT/oral because they are on atropine. Add multivitamins and correct electrolyte imbalance.
- Enteral feeding can be started when atropine is tapered and bowel sounds are heard, watching for RT returns.
- Catheterisation of bladder to prevent retention due to atropine
- IV pantoprazole to prevent stress ulcers.
- TPN as a last option
- Antibiotics as indicated: Avoid aminoglycosides as they may cause more paralysis.

Specific Treatment

Cholinergic toxicity: Reversed by atropine (1 amp=1 mL = 0.6 mg), also available as 100 mL injection (1 mL = 1 mg)

Initial: Atropine: 2–5 mg IV

Double the dose of IV atropine every 5 min to achieve adequate atropinization:
- Clear chest on auscultation/dryness of tongue and axillae
- Heart rate >80 beats/min, BP >90 mm of Hg
- Mydriasis
- Restlessness/delirium

Follow with continuous infusion of 10–20% per hour of the initial dose of atropine that was required to achieve atropinization.

Note

Continue till the patient is fully atropinised, and there is no sign of OP returning for 24–48 hours. Never stop atropine abruptly. It should be tapered slowly always, as the poison can return from fat depots.

Pralidoxime (to reactivate AChE)–(1 amp = 20 mL = 500 mg)

- It is important that pralidoxime be administered as soon as possible before permanent and irreversible aging occurs.
- Dose—IV bolus 30 mg/kg, mixed with normal saline and infused over slowly over 30 minutes.
- Followed by continuous infusion: 8 mg/kg per hour for 24–48 hr (WHO recommendation), Or
- Patients may be given 1–2 grams IV 8th hourly for 24–48 hr.
- It should be administered slowly over a period of one hour in 100–200 mL NS/5D
- Rapid infusion—can cause cardiac arrest, hypotension, neuromuscular blockade
- Duration: Till patient becomes asymptomatic, or at least as long as atropine is required

Seizures

- Benzodiazepines are used in case of seizures. Prophylactic dose (diazepam 10–20 mg IV) has shown to improve neurocognitive defects in OP poisoning.

- Prognosis:
  - Studies show that GCS of less than 13 points towards poor prognosis.
  - Age, comorbidities, delayed intervention lead to poor prognosis.

Delayed Neuropathy

- Occurs 1–3 weeks after ingestion
- Transient, painful "stocking-glove" paresthesias followed by a symmetrical motor polyneuropathy characterized by flaccid weakness of the lower extremities, which ascends to involve the upper extremities.
- Primarily affects distal muscle groups, but in severe neurotoxicity, proximal muscles groups may also be affected.

Carbamates

Bendiocarb/carbofuran/carbaryl/methomyl

Carbamates transiently and reversibly bind to and inhibit the cholinesterase enzyme. Regeneration of enzyme activity occurs within minutes to a few hours and involves rapid, spontaneous hydrolysis of the carbamate–cholinesterase bond.

Therefore, aging does not occur

Clinical features are the same as OP compounds, including muscarinic, nicotinic and CNS toxicity including rarely, seizures.

Differences from OP

- Milder course and better prognosis
- PAM not needed, and less severe toxicity
- Treat with atropine as given above.
- Diazepam for seizures.

Chapter

70

Paraquat Poisoning

Paraquat is a rapidly acting non selective herbicide, used commonly by farmers.

Toxic dose

Lethal dose 2–4 g (30 mL—two mouthfuls) of 20% concentrated paraquat.
10 mL causes serious organ damage

Mechanism of Action

1. Concentrated solutions (>20%): Corrosive injuries to mucous membrane and skin irritation
2. After rapid absorption, paraquat is concentrated inside cells where it undergoes redox cycling—leading to formation of free radicals like superoxide and hydroxyl anions
3. Cell death through lipid peroxidation, mitochondrial toxicity

Organs Affected

- GI tract corrosion
- Lung—ARDS and fibrosis
- Kidney—acute kidney injury
- Liver dysfunction
- Cardiac dysfunction

Clinical Features

***Mild poisoning:* <20 mg/kg** ingestion—usually recover.

- Pain and swelling of mouth and throat, followed by ulceration in 1–2 days
- Nausea, vomiting, diarrhea and pain abdomen.

Moderate poisoning: 20–40 mg/kg (2 target organs: Lung and kidney involved)

1–3 days: ARDS initially—pneumonitis

2–6 days: Renal failure, hepatic impairment and hypotension.

1–2 wk: Cough, hemoptysis, pleural effusion and pulmonary fibrosis.

Survival is possible, but majority of cases die within 2–3 weeks from pulmonary failure.

***Severe poisoning:* >40 mg/kg**

- Severe gastritis and gastroenteritis
- Massive fluid loss and electrolyte imbalance
- Rapid onset AKI

- Shock, severe metabolic acidosis death within hours.
- Pulmonary edema
- Convulsions
- Hepatic injury—uncommon and not cause of death
- Death from cardiogenic shock and multiorgan failure within 1–4 days.

Diagnosis

- History of intake associated with oral and gastric ulcers.
- Presence of AKI and ARDS
- Liver and renal function tests, chest X-ray, arterial blood gas, CBC are other useful investigations.

Paraquat levels in serum and urine: Dithionite test

Treatment

Emergency and supportive treatment

- Maintenance of airway, mechanical ventilation if needed.
- Correction of electrolyte disturbance
- Oxygen should not be administered unless hypoxia is confirmed, as oxygen stimulates superoxide radical formation and promotes oxidative stress.

Decontamination

- Remove contaminated clothes and wash exposed skin with soap and water. Irrigation of eyes with saline.
- Activated charcoal: 1–2 grams/kg with repeated doses every 1–2 hours.
- Gastric lavage is contraindicated due to the high likelihood of paraquat-induced corrosive injury

Treatment of Major Organ Dysfunction

ARDS

- Target pO_2 of around 60 mmHg in case the patient is hypoxic.
- *Oxygen should be given only in case of severe hypoxia as it acts as a substrate from which bipyridyls create harmful free radicals species.*

Renal failure: Hemodialysis

Pain Management

- Fentanyl: A bolus of 100 µg of fentanyl or infusion with 500 µg in 40 mL normal saline at 3–5 mL per hour in case the patient is on mechanical ventilation.
- Avoid NSAIDs in view of kidney injury.

Specific treatment

There is **no specific antidote** for paraquat poisoning.

Hemoperfusion (as soon as possible)

- Hemoperfusion can remove paraquat and has been recommended within 4 hours.
- Usually around 4–6 sessions are done each around 4 hours.
- Useful to limit lung injury.

Anti-inflammatory and Immunosuppressive Therapy

Steroids:

Dexamethasone 8 mg IV 8th hourly for the first 72 hours. This can be continued in tapering doses over 4–6 weeks, based on the patients lung condition.

Cyclophosphamide:

- Prehydration with 500 mL normal saline over 2 hours
- Followed by IV ranitidine 50 mg and IV ondansetron 4 mg injections 1 ampule each.
- Injection MESNA 400 mg IV infusion (to prevent hemorrhagic cystitis)
- Injection cyclophosphamide (5–15 mg/kg) given as an infusion in 500 mL NS over 2 hours.
- Injection MESNA 400 mg IV infusion
- Hydration with 500 mL normal saline

Note: *Combination of steroids and cyclophosphamide has shown no benefit*

Antioxidant therapy of doubtful value

N-acetyl cysteine

- 150 mg/kg stat followed by
- 50 mg/kg over 4 hours and then
- 100 mg/kg over 16 hours

Pain Management

- Fentanyl: A bolus of 100 μg of fentanyl or infusion with 500 μg in 40 mL normal saline at 3–5 mL per hour in case the patient is on mechanical ventilation.
- Avoid NSAIDs in view of kidney injury.

Prognosis

- Moderate–severe paraquat poisoning have poor prognosis.
- The mortality rates are still very high reaching around 50–60%.
- Higher serum lactate level is associated with poor prognosis.
- Most common causes of death would be hypoxia, shock, multiple organ dysfunction syndrome, ARDS and respiratory failure, which can occur even after week 2.
- Late complication—pulmonary fibrosis

Chapter

71

Rodenticide Poisoning

Content

- 3% yellow phosphorus. Available as a paste (Ratol) with 15 gm paste with net content of 450 mg of phosphorus.
- Others are zinc phosphide and aluminium phosphide.

Toxicity

- Toxic dose: More than 1 mg/kg of product

Mechanism of Toxicity

- Phosphorus—absorbed through the gastrointestinal tract.
- Converted into phosphine after ingestion, which acts as a protoplasmic toxin which inhibits various enzymes and protein synthesis, affecting the hepatic, gastrointestinal and cardiovascular systems.
- In the circulation, phosphorus binds to calcium and can cause hypocalcemia.

Clinical Manifestations

These can be divided into following phases

1. First 24 hours
   - Vomiting and diarrhea
   - Perioral and mucosal burns.

   Death in this stage is due to cardiac arrest or ventricular dysrhythmias in this phase.
2. 24–72 hours; asymptomatic phase
   - **Patient is deceptively asymptomatic**
   - May have an increase in bilirubin levels and liver enzymes—signifies deterioration.
3. More than 72 hours, dangerous phase
   - They can manifest with acute liver failure (ALF—very high liver enzymes and bilirubin), coagulopathy, hypotension, cardiac arrhythmias, and acute kidney injury
   - Most commonly affected organ is the liver.

Investigations

- Increases bilirubin, both direct and indirect
- AST and ALT can be more than 1000 IU/L
- Prolonged PT/INR—coagulopathy.

- Hypoglycemia
- Acute kidney injury with renal failure
- Confusion/psychosis/hallucinations
- Cardiac arrhythmias/myocarditis
- Hemolysis
- Cause of death in this phase is acute fulminant hepatitis with bleeding manifestations due to coagulopathy.

Management

Decontamination

- Gastric lavage with potassium permanganate is advised to remove ingested poison.
- Activated charcoal 1 gm/kg 6th hourly to decrease absorption.

Specific Treatment

There is no specific treatment. N-acetylcysteine has been tried with some success.

NAC 2 mL in 1 amp = 400 mg
N-acetylcysteine infusion can be started as early as possible

IV dose: 21 hours regimen

- Loading dose of 150 mg/kg in 100 mL 5% D over 1 hour
- Followed by 50 mg/kg in 500 mL 5% D for 4 hours
- Followed by 100 mg/kg in 1000 mL 5% D for the next 16 hours.

Oral dose: 72 hours regimen

- Loading dose: 140 mg/kg
- Maintenance dose: 70 mg/kg every 4 hours; repeat dose if emesis occurs within 1 hour of administration

Oral NAC can be continued till LFT normalizes.

Supportive Care

- Prevention of hepatic encephalopathy in early stages of poisoning with rifaximin 550 mg bd and lactulose 30 mL qid
- Fresh frozen plasma (4 units) can be used to control bleeding due to deranged coagulation parameters.
- If PT prolonged—Vitamin-K 10 mg IV q8th hourly for 3 days
- IV dextrose for hypoglycemia.

Liver Transplant

- In institutions where the facilities exist can be done in case of acute liver failure if the patient is deteriorating with the above care.
- Monitoring
- Liver enzymes (AST, ALT, ALT) along with PT/INR, APTT should be monitored daily.
- There is usually a sudden increase in liver enzymes on the 3rd day of consumption of the poison.

- Electrolytes such as potassium, calcium and phosphorus should be monitored with rapid correction on hypocalcemia or hypokalemia.

Prognosis

- The prognosis of the individual depends on the amount of poison taken.
- Small amount of poison usually is asymptomatic.
- Close observation and supportive management decreases the mortality rate in these individuals.

Aluminium Phosphide

- Inhalation causes irritation of nose, throat and lungs
- Ingestion of this causes myocarditis, and acute kidney injury
- Treatment : IV magnesium with monitoring of levels

Zinc Phosphide

- Oral ingestion: Same as ratol
- Causes ARDS, liver and kidney dysfunction
- Treatment is supportive.

Chapter

72

Paracetamol Poisoning

Most common cause of acute liver failure in the United States, United Kingdom, and Canada.

Toxic Doses

- >10 grams or 200 milligrams/kg as a single ingestion.

Mechanism of Toxicity

In overdose, acetaminophen is oxidized by the CYP450 system to a reactive metabolite, N-acetyl-p-benzoquinone imine (NAPQI). In paracetamol overdose, hepatic stores of glutathione decrease to <30% of normal, and NAPQI causes centrilobular hepatic necrosis.

Factors that increase the susceptibility to paracetamol-induced hepatotoxicity and acute liver failure:

- Age > 40 years
- Malnutrition or a fasting state
- Chronic liver disease/chronic alcohol use
- Pregnancy
- Concomitant use of other hepatotoxic medications: Isoniazid, rifampin, phenobarbital, statins.

Clinical Features

- Phase 1: First 24 hours after ingestion
  - Nonspecific symptoms—nausea, vomiting, abdominal pain and anorexia
- Phase 2: 24 – 72 hours after ingestion
  - Symptoms may improve or disappear
  - Right upper quadrant pain/tenderness
  - Liver function test: Elevated transaminases and bilirubin, prolonged prothrombin time (PT)
- Phase 3: 72 – 96 hours after ingestion (phase of maximal liver injury)
  - Nausea and vomiting reappear or worsen
  - Jaundice/coagulopathy/hepatic encephalopathy
  - Renal failure/metabolic acidosis
  - Central nervous system symptoms: Confusion, somnolence and coma

- Phase 4: 96 hours—14 days after ingestion
    - Patient may start improving and have full recovery within 3 months or
    - Patient may progress to multiorgan failure and death.

Investigations

- Serum paracetamol levels:
    - Measure as soon as possible.
- Paracetamol levels in blood: >300 microgrms/mL should be considered dangerous, and start treatment
- Basic investigations—CBC, RFT, LFT, amylase and lipase
- Deranged LFTs: Typically, present 24–72 hours post-ingestion
    - Increased ALT: can be >1,000 units/L
    - Increased AST: can be >1,000 units/L
    - Increased alkaline phosphatase, increased bilirubin
    - Prolonged prothrombin time (PT), elevated INR
- Other blood tests to assess the severity of an overdose: Part of the King's College Hospital (KCH) criteria
    - Arterial pH
    - Serum creatinine
    - Blood lactate levels
    - Phosphate levels

Management

- Supportive therapy
    - Gastrointestinal decontamination with activated charcoal (1 g/kg) in divided doses if the patient presents within 1–2 hours of ingestion
    - Hemodialysis in patients with a massive overdose
    - **Antidote therapy:** N-acetylcysteine (NAC) (available 2 mL ampoules 200 mg in 1 mL)
    - Begin NAC within 8 hour post-ingestion mark (most effective).

Indications

- Acute overdose
- If time of ingestion is <8 hours, serum acetaminophen concentration is high
- If > 8 hours
    - Immediately begin empiric therapy
- Unknown time of ingestion
    - Initiate empiric NAC immediately;
    - Discontinue if acetaminophen concentration is undetectable and LFTs are within normal limits.

Dosing

- Intravenous 21 hour regimen: Dosing in adults
- Loading dose: 150 mg/kg in 100 mL 5% D over 1 hour

- Followed by 50 mg/kg in 500 mL 5% D over 4 hours
- Followed by 100 mg/kg in 1,000 mL 5% D over 16 hours
- **Oral administration:** 72 hours
- Alternative to the IV formulation in patients at increased risk for anaphylaxis with IV administration and those with initially low serum paracetamol levels (<150 μg/mL)
- Loading dose: 140 mg/kg
- Followed by: 70 mg/kg orally every 4 hours for 18 total doses
    - Duration of treatment

Treatment beyond typical protocol duration is indicated in patients with:

- Evidence of hepatotoxicity (i.e. elevated AST and ALT)
- Positive predictors of poor prognosis (e.g. decreased pH; increased phosphate, lactate, or creatinine levels; increased prothrombin time/INR)
- Persistent serum paracetamol levels detected by laboratory testing

Indications for stopping NAC treatment:

- Serum paracetamol level is <10 μg/mL
- Serum AST and ALT are not elevated higher than the reference range/not increasing.
- No signs or symptoms of hepatic dysfunction
- INR ≤1.3
- Indications for liver transplant:
    - For patients who progress to acute liver failure despite treatment with NAC
    - King's College Hospital criteria is most widely used prognostic criteria to determine need for liver transplant

List for transplant if

- Arterial pH <7.3 after adequate fluid resuscitation

All these occur within 24 hours

- Creatinine > 3.2mg/dL and all else.
- INR >6.5 (prothrombin time >100 seconds)
- Grade III/IV encephalopathy
- Arterial blood lactate levels (modified King's College Hospital criteria)
    - 31.5 mg/dL before adequate fluid resuscitation
    - 27 mg/dL after adequate fluid resuscitation

Chapter

73

Barbiturate Poisoning

Fatal dose: 6–10 grams of phenobarbital

Clinical Features (Table 73.1)

Table 73.1: Degree of poisoning

Severity	Dose of phenobarbital consumed	Features
Mild	<2 g	Patient is conscious and oriented Nil intervention required
Moderate	2–5 g	Patient is stuporous Pupils reacting Reflexes and vital signs normal
Severe	5–10 g	Deep coma/hypotension Hypothermia/ARDS/skin blisters

Investigation

- ABG
- Blood urea, serum creatinine and electrolytes
- Gas chromatography/mass spectrometry for identification and confirmation of presence of barbiturates
  - Blood levels >60–80 mg/L are usually associated with coma
  - Blood levels >150–200 mg/L with severe hypotension

MANAGEMENT

There is no specific antidote. Treatment is mainly supportive.

1. Establish a patent airway
   - Start oxygen
   - Intubate and ventilate if required
2. Establish an IV line
3. Elevate foot end of the bed (if BP is low)/start IV fluids/inotropes
4. Gastric lavage (using a stomach tube)
   - Useful if the patient is admitted early
   - Activated charcoal 1 gm/kg in divided doses
5. Inj. pantoprazole—to avoid stress ulcers/40 mg IV q12 h
6. Forced alkaline diuresis.

- Urinary alkalinization enhances the clearance of phenobarbital and primidone
- One cycle =
  - 1 litre DNS/1 litre NS with 20 mEq KCl +100 mL HCO_3
  - Inj. frusemide 40 mg IV
- Cycle to be repeated every 2–4 hours
- Maintain urine output at 300 mL/hour.
- Taper off cycle over 24–48 hr

7. Dialysis indications
   - Severely intoxicated patients
   - Oliguria
   - These are useful for only phenobarbital poisoning

Chapter

74

Beta-Blocker Toxicity

Complications of beta-blocker poisoning arise from excessive beta adrenergic blockade. It can also occur due to their pro-arrhythmic activity.

Clinical Features

Dizziness, nausea, altered mental status seizures and coma

On examination:

- Bradycardia and hypotension.
- Ventricular arrhythmias can be seen with acebutolol, propranolol, s
- Bronchospasm/respiratory depression
- Hypoglycemia—uncommon

Laboratory Findings

- ECG to look for bradycardia, PR prolongation, QT prolongation. In severe poisoning, any bradycardia can progress to asystole.
- Hyperkalemia
- Hypoglycemia
- Renal function tests, serum calcium levels.
- Calcium to be monitored 6th hourly in the case of calcium administration.
- Hourly glucose needs to be monitored in case insulin/glucose treatment is used.

Diagnosis

- History and clinical findings.
- Other causes for bradycardia need to be ruled out such as calcium channel blocker poisoning, digoxin toxicity, cholinergic agent (organophosphates) toxicity.

Management

General measures

- Activated charcoal: Give a single dose of activated charcoal (1 g/kg, up to 50 g maximum) to all patients who present within 2 hours of ingestion, unless contraindicated.
- Whole bowel irrigation with polyethylene glycol solution at 2 L/hour in adults, until clear rectal effluent, can be tried after a large ingestion of an extended-release product.

Specific therapy

Note

- In case of mildly symptomatic patients, fluids and atropine are used initially and then the next line of treatment is used in case of a lack of response.
- Time to check for lack of responsiveness of a treatment modality is 15 minutes.

If severe: use all these modalities

1. Glucagon:

- First line of therapy. Prolonged treatment causes tachyphylaxis.
- Initial 5 mg IV bolus over 1 minute. Recheck BP and pulse after 10–15 minutes. Repeat bolus in case of no increase.
- If there is a response to the second bolus, start infusion at 2–5 mg per hour.
- Goal of MAP is 60 mmHg.

2. Glucose-insulin therapy

- As per treatment of hyperkalemia (refer to the chapter on this topic)

3. Calcium

- 10 mL of 10% calcium chloride over 10 minutes slow IV via central line. May be given as frequently as every 8th hourly, or 30 mL of 10% calcium gluconate through a peripheral line can be given.
- The recommended dose of 10% calcium gluconate is 0.6 mL/kg given over 5 to 10 minutes, followed by a continuous infusion of 0.6 to 1.5 mL/kg per hour.

4. Vasopressors:

- Adrenaline started at 1 µg/minute can be given to raise the MAP to 60 mm of Hg.

5. Intravenous lipid emulsion (20% solution)

- Beneficial in the treatment of it from lipophilic β-blockers-propranolol and carvedilol
- Bolus: 1.5 mL/kg over 1 minute, followed by
- Infusion: 0.25 mL/kg per minute

6. Additional intervention:

- Sodium bicarbonate for QRS prolongation—1–2 mEq/kg IV bolus followed by 150 mEq in 350 mL 5% D at 125 mL/hr
- Magnesium for ventricular arrhythmia—2 g IV bolus
- Hemodialysis: Effective for atenolol intoxication, and should be considered when renal function is severely impaired
- Transvenous cardiac pacing for profound bradycardia
- Intra-aortic balloon pump for refractory hypotension
- Extracorporeal membrane oxygenation: For patients with severe ingestions who do not respond to standard therapy

Chapter

75

Tricyclic Antidepressants (TCA) Overdose

Commonly used antidepressants.

Mechanism

- Inhibition of presynaptic neurotransmitter reuptake (norepinephrine and serotonin).
- Antagonism of central and peripheral muscarinic acetylcholine receptors

Pharmacokinetics

- Absorbed from gastrointestinal tract
- Time taken to reach maximum plasma concentration-2–8 hours
- Metabolized by liver—active metabolites can persist in the plasma for 12–24 hours.
- Excretion—70% inactive components by kidney

Toxic Dose

- Life-threatening symptoms: If >10 mg/kg in adults, and fatalities, with ingestions of >1 gram total dose.

Clinical Features

Neurologic

- Sedation, coma and seizures
- Delirium and hallucinations (anticholinergic effect)

Cardiac

- Tachycardia, conduction abnormalities, VF and VT(4%—rare)
- Most common cause of death is refractory hypotension.

Anticholinergic

- Dilated pupils, dry mouth, ileus, urinary retention, increased muscle tone.

Diagnosis

Tricyclic antidepressant toxicity is diagnosed using a combination of four criteria:

- History of exposure
- Clinical symptomatology
- Characteristic ECG findings
- Positive cyclic antidepressant urine drug screen results

1. ECG.
   - Prolonged QRS > 100 milliseconds (correlates with incidence of seizure and VT)
   - R to S ratio >0.7 in aVR
   - R wave in aVR >3 mm
2. Quantitative tests in serum and qualitative tests in urine may help with the diagnosis.

Management

Initial resuscitation

- Airway: Patients with TCA poisoning might require early intubation for airway protection
- Breathing: Oxygen therapy, ventilatory support
- Circulation: Boluses of crystalloids for hypotension
- Activated charcoal: Dose of 1g/kg (50 g maximum) if the patient presents within 2 hours of poisoning.
- Conduction abnormalities-
  - Sodium bicarbonate: (Reduces active form of drug)
    - 2–3 meq/kg IV push (up to 150 mEq) and reassess QRS interval.
    - If QRS narrowing begins, continue infusion with 150 mEq sodium bicarbonate in 500 mL 5% D at 125 mL/hr.
    - Target pH on ABG should be 7.5–7.55.
  - Temporary pacemaker: For bradyarrhythmias

Refractory hypotension

- Vasopressors are used in hypotension refractory to bicarbonate and fluids.
- Norepinephrine is the preferred vasopressor
- Hypertonic saline: Controversial when hypotension is refractory. 100 mL IV bolus of 3% NaCl can be used and checked for response, every 10 minutes a maximum of 300 mL is used.
- High dose glucagon up to 10 mg: Due to inotropic and chronotropic effects on myocardial tissue.

Refractory arrhythmias: Magnesium (1–2 g over 15 minutes) can be used in addition to bicarbonate.

- Lignocaine, bolus dose (1–1.5 mg/kg IV), followed by an infusion (1–4 mg/minute)

Others

- Seizures: Usually self-limiting. Benzodiazepines are treatment of choice. Phenytoin is contraindicated.
- Physostigmine is contraindicated to treat anticholinergic effects as it is associated with cardiac arrest in TCA poisoning.
- Intravenous lipid emulsion therapy: For severe tricyclic overdose, especially with amitriptyline and clomipramine.

Prognosis

- Severe toxicity has poor prognosis due to refractory hypotension and arrhythmias.
- QRS duration predicts ventricular arrhythmias.

Chapter

76

Opioid Poisoning

Includes toxicity caused by:

- Short-acting opioids:
  - Morphine sulfate, fentanyl and fentanyl analogues, oxycodone, hydrocodone, codeine, heroin
- Longer-acting and delayed-release opioids
  - Extended-release morphine sulfate, methadone and oxymorphone
- Opioid receptor agonist-antagonist drugs:
  - Pentazocine, butorphanol, nalbuphine and buprenorphine

Clinical Features

- History of opioid use or abuse
- Acetaminophen co-ingestion is common
- Respiratory depression/Central nervous system depression: Drowsiness and coma
- **Miosis**
- **Other features:**
  - Bradycardia/hypotension/hypothermia
  - *Skin examination:* Evidence of fentanyl patch, needle track marks
  - *Seizures:* Tramadol, dextromethorphan, and meperidine may cause seizures by lowering the seizure threshold
  - Pulmonary edema
- Death usually results from apnea or pulmonary aspiration

Investigations

- Urine toxicology:
  - Positive toxicology results may indicate presence of opioids. However, toxicology screening may be falsely negative if opioid is fentanyl, methadone or oxycodone.
- ECG—for QT prolongation
- ABG—type 2 respiratory failure

Management

- ***Decontamination:***
  - Activated charcoal
    - 1 gram/kg orally or via gastric tube if ingestion within 2 hours
  - Removal of fentanyl patch, if present

- *Airway and breathing:*
    - Restore respiration using a bag valve mask until naloxone can be administered
    - Advanced airway—rarely required
- *Specific treatment:*
    - **Naloxone hydrochloride**—reversal agent
    - **Reversal proves the diagnosis**
    - Dosing: 0.4 to 2 mg IV, IM, or SC every 2 to 3 minutes as needed. Total dose of 10 mg
    - Large doses (10–20 mg) may be needed for codeine, fentanyl derivatives
    - Long-acting opioid exposure may require naloxone infusion for persistent or recurrent respiratory depression—only if the patient responded to the initial naloxone bolus (off label)
        - Dose: 0.25–6.25 mg/hr IV
        - To calculate the naloxone continuous infusion dose, determine the "wake-up dose" and administer two-thirds of that dose per hour by IV infusion.
    - Other routes of administration: Intranasal, endotracheal tube, nebulized
    - Note: Do not administer orally because it has high first-pass metabolism rate
    - Observe patient for 4 to 6 hours after the last dose of naloxone
    - Naloxone may precipitate withdrawal symptoms such as chills, vomiting, diarrhea, anxiety, irritability, and restlessness.

Chapter

77

Methemoglobinemia

- Methemoglobin is a form of hemoglobin that is oxidized(ferrous to ferric form).
- Hence it binds irreversibly to oxygen and cannot deliver oxygen to the tissues.

Types

1. Congenital methemoglobinemia presents with cyanosis but is asymptomatic. It is a rare entity.
2. Acquired methemoglobinemia—mostly drug induced and can be severe depending on the proportion of methemoglobin.

Acquired Methemoglobinemia

Acute acquired methemoglobinemia can cause severe hypoxia and death.

Causes

Drugs

- Amino salicylic acid/sulfonamides
- Clofazimine/dapsone
- Chloroquine/primaquine
- Nitroglycerin/methylene blue (in high doses in people with G6PD deficiency)
- Chemicals and dyes—aniline dyes/antifreeze/benzene derivatives
- Herbicides and larvicides poisoning
- Copper sulphate poisoning

Symptoms

Depends on the methemoglobin levels

- 0–3% normal range
- 3–12% clinically detectable cyanosis
- 3–20% asymptomatic unless there is a pre-existing condition
- 20–50% fatigue, mild dyspnea, lethargy
- 50–70% respiratory depression, altered sensorium, coma, seizures
- >70% fatal

Clinical Clues

- Presence of cyanosis with low O_2 saturation by probe, but normal PaO_2 on ABG
- Saturation may not improve even with oxygen administration
- Pulse oximetry is unreliable and shows false values.

Management

Acquired methemoglobinemia

Evaluation

- Observation of color of blood: Chocolate brown color
- Arterial blood gas shows normal paO_2
- Methemoglobin levels (>5% is abnormal)
- G6PD levels—methylene blue should not be administered in G6PD deficiency

Differential diagnosis

- Carbon monoxide poisoning
- Sulfhemoglobin poisoning

Initial Management

Acute toxicity with levels >30% is an emergency

- Discontinuation of offending drug
- Supportive care:
  - IV hydration and inotropes for hypotension
  - Ventilation if required
  - Anti-epileptic medication if warranted

Specific Therapy

1. Methylene blue

- Mild toxicity (20–30%)
  - Start with 1 mg/kg IV given over 5 minutes
  - Dose can be repeated after one hour if methemoglobin levels are rising or has not decreased to less than 20%
- Moderate to severe toxicity (30–50% or patients with severe symptoms)
  - 1–2 mg/kg is given IV over 5 minutes
  - Dose can be repeated after one hour if methemoglobin levels are rising or has not decreased to less than 20%
  - More than 2–3 doses (or >7 mg/kg) is avoided as it can cause hemolysis even in individuals with normal G6PD
- Optimum dose of methylene blue is unknown
- Clinical response usually occurs within 10–60 minutes
- Contraindications
  - G6PD deficiency
  - Selective serotonin reuptake inhibitors (SSRI) use

2. Ascorbic acid

- Used when MB is unavailable
- Dose—300 mg IV stat

- Improvement might take 1–3 days
- Side effects—renal failure in high doses

Other Therapies

- Cimetidine:
  - In dapsone—induced methemoglobinemia.
  - Blocks hepatic metabolism of dapsone into active metabolites that contribute to MetHb formation.
- Exchange transfusion:
  - In patients with severe methemoglobinemia, if methylene blue is contraindicated (e.g. G6PD deficiency) or has not been effective.
- Hyperbaric oxygen:
  - Can supply sufficient oxygen independently of hemoglobin.
  - May be useful in extremely serious cases that do not respond rapidly to antidotal treatment.

Congenital methemoglobinemia

Infants with cytochrome B_5 reductase deficiency are treated with

- Methylene blue 100–300 mg PO per day, Or
- Ascorbic acid 1000 mg tid

Chapter

78

Carbon Monoxide Poisoning

Sources

The common sources of carbon monoxide poisoning are fire related smoke inhalation.

Others

- Poorly functioning heating systems
- Improperly vented fuel-burning devices: Kerosene heaters, charcoal grills
- Motor vehicles operating in poorly ventilated areas

Pathophysiology

Carbon monoxide (CO) diffuses rapidly across the pulmonary capillary membrane and binds to the iron moiety of heme with approximately 240 times the affinity of oxygen, causing left shift of oxygen hemoglobin dissociation curve and poor oxygen delivery.

Carbon monoxide can also interfere with molecules such as cytochromes, NADPH reductase which impair oxidative phosphorylation at a mitochondrial level.

Clinical Features

a. Major toxicity symptoms:
   - Loss of consciousness, confusion and Seizures,
   - Rarely non-cardiogenic pulmonary edema.

b. Minor toxicity symptoms:
   - Headache, dizziness, vomiting and nausea
   - Acute myocardial injury is possible in patients with carbon monoxide poisoning which increases mortality.

c. Delayed neuropsychiatric syndrome:
   - Occurs in 40% of carbon monoxide poisoning. Can occur between 3 and 240 days.
   - Characterized by cognitive deficits, personality changes, movement disorders, and focal neurologic deficits.

Diagnosis

- History and physical examination: Features suggestive of carbon monoxide poisoning.
- SpO_2 probes show falsely normal saturation, but arterial oxygen is low. This is called the pulse oximetry gap. *Check oxygenation using arterial blood gas.*

- CO level with CO-oximetry of arterial or venous blood can be checked—gold standard
- Definitive diagnosis: COHb concentration >20%
- Suspect CO poisoning if COHb >10% + clinical findings
- Lactic acidosis can occur in severe poisoning.
- ECG: Measure cardiac biomarkers in patients ≥65 and in patients with ischemic symptoms.
- CT brain in patients with altered mental status.

Treatment

Initial management

- Remove from the source of poisoning.
- Immediate access to high flow oxygen (irrespective of oxygen saturation) using non-rebreathing mask.
- Noninvasive ventilation using 100% oxygen can also be given. This should be continued till carboxy hemoglobin falls below 10%.
- Comatose patients and patients with altered mental status can be considered for early intubation and anti-cerebral edema measures.

Hyperbaric oxygen (HBO) therapy:

- Indications
  - CO level >25 percent
  - CO level >20 percent in pregnant patient
  - Loss of consciousness
  - Severe metabolic acidosis (pH <7.1)
  - Evidence of end-organ ischemia—ECG changes, altered mental status
- Evidence suggests that use of HBO within 6 hours of poisoning can help in prevention of delayed neuropsychiatric syndrome. Unlikely to be useful 24 hours after poisoning.

Prognosis

- Mild to moderate poisoning: Recover with high flow oxygen.
- In case of severe poisoning: Requiring prolonged intubation or patients with hypoxic damage to the brain, supportive care is the only alternative.

Chapter

79

Methanol Poisoning

Toxic dose

- Minimal toxic dose: 1 gram/kg or about 100 mL in an adult.

Clinical Features

- 0 to 6 hours:
  - Patient may be asymptomatic
  - Confusion/ataxia
  - Formaldehyde odor on breath
  - Abdominal pain

  6 to 12 hours:
  - Malaise/abdominal pain, vomiting
  - Headache/visual manifestations: Hyperemia of optic disc, 'snow vision,' and blindness
- More than 12 hours:
  - High anion gap metabolic acidosis
  - Cerebral edema
  - Hyperglycemia
  - Shock/multiorgan failure

Laboratory Investigations

- Elevated osmolal gap—early
- High anion gap metabolic acidosis—later due to its metabolite formate.
- Blood methanol levels (by gas chromatography): Levels >50 mg/dL indicates serious poisoning.
- Serum formate levels—consistent with methanol poisoning;
- Urea, creatinine, electrolytes, glucose, amylase, and ABG should be monitored every 4 hours.

Treatment

Supportive therapy:

- Protect the airway and assisted ventilation, as needed

- Sodium bicarbonate 1 to 2 mEq/kg intravenously for metabolic acidosis bolus followed by infusion of 1–3 mEq/kg $NaHCO_3$ in 1 L D5W to run at 200 to 250 mL/hour for patients with pH below 7.3.

Note: 1 mL of 8.4% sodium bicarbonate = 1 mEq)

- Adequate fluids and hydration.
- Thiamine, pyridoxine, and multivitamin supplementation—in patients with suspected alcohol abuse disorder
- Anticonvulsants to treat seizures
- Note: Gastric decontamination techniques usually ineffective due to rapid absorption of methanol.

Hemodialysis

- Used in conjunction with antidote therapy
- Indications:
  - Blood methanol concentration >50 mg/dL (>25 mg/dL in some centers)
  - Serum formate level >20 mg/dL
  - Visual changes, seizures and clinical deterioration despite intensive supportive therapy
  - Significant refractory metabolic acidosis and electrolyte abnormalities

Antidote therapy

- Indications: If the patient has a history of ingesting more than 0.4 mL/kg of 100% methanol with the following conditions:
- Blood methanol level > 20 mg/dL
- Osmolar gap not accounted for by other factors
- Symptomatic or acidotic with increased anion gap and/or hyperemia of the optic disc

1. Ethanol therapy

- *Loading dose:* 10 mL/kg of 10% ethanol IV in D5W be given over 60 minutes
- *Maintenance dose:* 1 mL/kg/h of 10% ethanol IV. This dose may need to be increased to 2 mL/kg/h in heavy drinkers

2. Fomepizole therapy (blocks alcohol dehydrogenase)

- Loading dose: 15 mg/kg (0.015 mL/kg) IV
- Maintenance dose:
  - 10 mg/kg (0.01 mL/kg) every 12 hours for 4 doses
  - Then 15 mg/kg every 12 hours until the ethylene glycol levels are less than 20 mg/dL
- The solution is prepared by being mixed with 100 mL of 0.9% saline or 5% dextrose
- Dose adjustment is required for patients being taken up for hemodialysis

Other

- **Leucovorin:** 1 mg/kg up to 50 mg IV is administered every 6 hours, to enhance formate metabolism to carbon dioxide and water.

Common poisoning and overdose		
Substance	**Clinical features**	**Immediate treatment plan**
Acids Sulphuric acid Nitric acid Hydrochloric acid	• Oral, esophageal and gastric erosions, ulcers and bleeding • Laryngeal edema	No specific treatment • Gastric lavage with soft tube if seen within 90 minutes • Irrigate and wash oral cavity, eyes and skin with flowing water • Milk of magnesia to neutralize acid • Morphine for pain • IV dexamethasone 4 mg IV stat and 8th hourly for laryngeal edema • Antibiotics
Alkalis	• Oral, esophageal and gastric burns • GI bleeding • Aspiration • Laryngeal edema	• Irrigate and wash oral cavity, eyes and skin with flowing water • Gastric lavage with soft tube if seen within 90 minutes • Glucocorticoids for laryngeal edema
Aluminium sulfide (a fungicide)	• Headache • Dizziness • Convulsion • Coma • Hypotension • Arrhythmia • Myocarditis • Respiratory failure • Renal failure • Hepatitis	• Gastric lavage • Magnesium sulphate 1 gm IV infusion over one hour every 3–6 hourly for 3–6 days
Yellow oleander Cerebra Thevetia and odollam	• Digitalis like action • Atrioventricular blocks and VT • Bradycardia • Hypotension	• Stomach wash • 1/6 molar sodium lactate and glucose • Antiarrhythmic drugs like amiodarone, phenytoin, lidocaine • Atropine for bradycardia • Inotropic support
Copper sulphate	• Vomiting • Abdominal pain • Diarrhea • Hypotension • Renal failure • Jaundice • Hemolysis • Coma	• Gastric lavage with 1% potassium ferro cyanide • Demulcents • Penicillamine 1–2 grams in 2 divided doses IV • Hemodialysis • Blood transfusion

Contd.

Common poisoning and overdose (Contd)		
Cyanide	• Bitter almond smell • Rapid onset action • Respiratory depression/ apnoea • Seizures/myoclonic jerks • Lock jaw • Tachycardia followed by bradycardia, arrhythmias • Hypotension	• 100% oxygen/ET tube insertion and mechanical ventilation • Amyl nitrate 0.2 mL inhaled form repeat every minute till sodium nitrite infusion is initiated • Sodium nitrite (10 mL of 3%) IV injection followed by 50 mL 25% sodium thiosulphate OR • 2 ampoules of 1.5% dicobalt tetracemate IV followed by 20 mL of 50% glucose IV over 1 minute
Diazepam	• Respiratory depression • Hypoventilation • Hypotension • Coma	• Gastric lavage • Activated charcoal • Respiratory support, oxygen, ET intubation, mechanical ventilation • Vasopressors • Specific antidote is flumezanil IV 0.2 – 0.5 mg at 1 minute interval until effect is seen or maximum dose of 3–5 mg • Flumazenil can cause convulsions if patient has co-ingested TCA or has benzodiazepine dependence • Diazepam is NOT dialyzable • Amiodarone, phenytoin and lidocaine for arrhythmias • Magnesium sulfate infusion for resistant arrhythmias
Ethanol	• CNS suppression • Delirium • Suppression of respiration • Hypoglycemia • Hypotension	• Hemodialysis if severe • Thiamine 500–1000 mg IV stat followed by IV glucose
Heavy metals Gold Mercury Arsenic Lead	• Liver and renal failure • Skin and mucosal changes • Bone marrow suppression	• Dimercaprol (BAL) • 3–5 mg/kg 4th hourly total 400–800 mg on day 1 • 200–400 mg on day 2 and 3 • 100–200 mg on day 4 and 5 • In case of lead: Sodium calcium edetate for 2–7 days • Penicillamine 1–2 grams PO daily in 4 divided doses
Heparin	• Bleeding (internal or external)	• 1 mg protamine sulfate to neutralize 100 units of heparin

Contd.

Common poisoning and overdose (Contd)		
Hydrocarbons Kerosene Petrol Organic solvents	• Vomiting • Aspiration • Hypoxia/dyspnea • Altered sensorium	• Stomach wash • ET tube and mechanical ventilation • Oxygen
Isoniazid	• Seizure • Delirium/psychosis	• Vit B_6 (pyridoxine) 5 grams slow IV over 5 – 30 minutes infusion
Lithium	• Drowsiness • Polyuria • Diarrhea • Hypernatremia • Ataxia	• Gastric lavage • Activated charcoal is of no use • Sodium polystyrene sulfonate used as an adsorbent • Diazepam/midazolam for convulsions • Hydration and correction of electrolytes • Hemodialysis if serum lithium level is > 5 mmol/L
Oxalic acid	• Severe irritation and burns of nose, throat, and respiratory tract. • Inhalation of oxalic acid dust or vapour can also cause protein in the urine, nosebleed, ulceration of the mucous membranes, headache, nervousness, cough, vomiting, emaciation, back pain and weakness	• Stomach wash • Calcium carbonate • Demulcents • Calcium gluconate sow IV infusion
Naphthalene balls (naphthalene or para-dichlorobenzene)	• Headaches, nausea, dizziness, vomiting diarrhea, fever, abdominal pain • Severe hemolysis in people with G6PD deficiency state	• Supportive and symptomatic care
Phenol (carbolic acid)	• Delirium • Convulsion • Coma	• IV Na HCO_3 7.5% 50 mL IV stat if CNS effects are observed
Dettol/Lysol (chloroxylenol (C_8H_9ClO), pine oil, isopropanol, castor oil, soap)	• Central nervous system depression • Corrosion of the oral mucosa, larynx and the gastrointestinal tract	• 30 mL/kg of oral liquid paraffin • Forced alkaline diuresis • Hemodialysis
Phenothiazine	• CNS suppression • Coma • Hypotension • Arrhythmias • EPS • Hyperpyrexia (NMS)	• Gastric lavage • Diphenhydramine for EPS • Normal saline infusion and vasopressors • Treatment of arrhythmias

Contd.

Common poisoning and overdose (Contd)		
Salicylates	• Confusion • Convulsion • GI bleeding • Vomiting • Metabolic acidosis • Renal failure • Pulmonary edema	• Gastric lavage • Activated charcoal 25 grams • Adequate hydration • Sodium bicarbonate infusion • Forced alkaline diuresis • Hemodialysis in severe cases
Strychnine	• Convulsions • Respiratory depression	• Gastric lavage with 1: 10,000 potassium permanganate solution • Benzodiazepine for seizure • Supportive measures
Theophylline	• Nausea • Vomiting • Delirium • Convulsions	• Gastric lavage • Activated charcoal • Supportive care • Hemodialysis/hemoperfusion • Adenosine for SVTs • Amiodarone/lidocaine for VT • Benzodiazepine for seizure (avoid phenytoin)
Coumarin derivatives/ Warfarin	• Bleeding tendency • Internal and external bleed • PT INR prolongation	• Stomach wash • Vit K 10 mg IV q8 h up to 50 mg • Fresh frozen plasma if active bleeding present

Chapter

80

Alcohol Withdrawal

Clinical Features

Suspect alcohol withdrawal in any patient who is alcohol dependent and has stopped or reduced their alcohol intake within hours or days of presentation

Table 80.1: Features of alcohol withdrawal

Stage	Time since stopping alcohol	Clinical features
Stage 1: Minor withdrawal symptoms	6–12 hours	Tremors, insomnia, irritability, anxiety, sweating, anorexia, nausea, vomiting
Stage 2: Withdrawal seizures	May begin as early as 2 hours after stopping alcohol 24–48 hours;	Usually generalized tonic-clonic seizures
Stage 3: Alcoholic hallucinosis	12–48 hours	Auditory, visual, or tactile hallucinations
Stage 4: Alcohol withdrawal delirium (delirium tremens)	Usually occurs 3–5 days after stopping; up to 14 days	Hallucinations (usually visual), disorientation, tachycardia, hypertension, agitation, diaphoresis, low-grade fever

Differential Diagnosis

- Hepatic encephalopathy
- Metabolic: Hypoglycemia
- Psychosis

Diagnosis

- Withdrawal is a clinical diagnosis and a diagnosis of exclusion
- To evaluate for concurrent problems/rule out differential diagnosis
  - Complete blood count, urea, creatinine and electrolyte levels, liver function tests, coagulation tests, blood glucose level, thyroid function tests
  - Blood alcohol level
  - Urine and/or serum drug screen
  - Neuroimaging: If possibility of head trauma/other CNS abnormalities
  - Lumbar puncture if CNS infection is suspected

- Evaluate for reasons leading to sudden cessation of alcohol intake, such as precipitating illness
- Revised clinical institute withdrawal assessment for alcohol (CIWA-Ar)—May be used to assess severity of withdrawal and to guide treatment

Treatment

- **Supportive care**
  - IV fluids and correction of electrolyte abnormalities
  - Nutritional supplementation: Thiamine—100 mg IV 8th hourly, and multivitamin
  - Treat hypoglycemia, if present (Note: Administer thiamine prior to glucose)
  - Treat co-existing complications
- **Benzodiazepines**
  - May reduce alcohol withdrawal symptoms, seizures, and recurrent seizures
  - For patients with alcohol withdrawal and with CIWA-Ar score > 8–10
  - Minor alcohol withdrawal symptoms/alcoholic hallucinosis
    - In patients with no hepatic impairment, delirium, or dementia and are able to tolerate oral medication: Long-acting oral benzodiazepine such as diazepam 10–20 mg or chlordiazepoxide 25–100 mg, which can be repeated hourly till patient becomes quiet.
    - In patients with hepatic impairment, delirium, or dementia, or those who cannot tolerate oral medication: Short-acting benzodiazepine such as lorazepam (2–4 mg IV every 15–20 minutes, until the appropriate sedation is achieved)
  - In case of alcohol withdrawal seizures
    - Lorazepam 4 mg intravenously
    - A second dose after 10 minutes if seizures continue
  - For delirium tremens
    - If oral intake is possible: Tablet lorazepam 2–4 mg q8 h
    - If symptoms persist or oral medication is declined: Intravenous lorazepam 2–4 mg every 15–20 minutes
    - Goal: To achieve and then maintain light somnolence
    - For mild withdrawal: Oral lorazepam 2 mg 0-0-1
- **Second-line agents for seizures/delirium tremens:**
  - Phenobarbital
  - Propofol
- **Other anticonvulsants**
  - Avoid other anticonvulsants (e.g. levetiracetam, phenytoin, valproate, carbamazepine) for treatment or prophylaxis of seizures

  Antipsychotics: Haloperidol, olanzapine
- As adjunct to benzodiazepines for agitation or cognitive disturbance
- Avoid routine use of antipsychotics

- Lower seizure threshold/have anticholinergic effects such as tachycardia and worsening hypertension
- Mask symptoms of worsening withdrawal
- Increase risk of respiratory complications

- Others:
  - Clonidine or a beta blocker (e.g. atenolol): May be considered; As adjuncts to benzodiazepines in patients with persistent cardiac adrenergic symptoms
  - Alcohol de-addiction

Alcohol de-addiction

- Counselling
- Acamprol 333 mg 2-2-2 for 1 month to decrease craving

Chapter

81

Snake Bite

Clinical Features

History of snake bite

Local tissue inflammation can present as:

- Fang marks
- Pain/bleeding at the site of bite
- Swelling/blisters of the affected limb

Viper bites: Local reaction, usually severe and evident in a few minutes.

Cobra bites: Less local reaction. May be delayed up to 24 hours

Occult bite

- Usually seen with krait bite
- Fang marks not present

Systemic effects:

- Coagulopathy
- Neurological effects
- Renal failure
- Hemolysis

Coagulopathy features (viper bite)

- Epistaxis
- Gingival oozing
- Bleeding from venipuncture site
- Ecchymoses and bruising
- Hematuria, malena and hematemesis.

Neurological (cobra and krait)—due to neuromuscular junction involvement--

5 Ds: **D**yspnea, **d**ysphonia, **d**ysarthria, **d**iplopia, **d**ysphagia
2 Ps: **P**tosis, **p**aralysis

Chronological order

Furrowing of forehead—ptosis–diplopia–dysarthria–dysphonia–dyspnoea

Bedside tests of impending respiratory failure
① Single breath count → Numbers counted during exhalation (up to 40)

② Breath holding time → breath held in inspiration (> 45 sec is normal)
③ Ability to complete one sentence in one breath

Renal

- Patients can also present with hypotension, shock, decreased urine output and renal failure due to rhabdomyolysis.

Hemolysis

- Hemolysis part of DIC

Investigations

- Hb and peripheral smear—for hemolysis
- platelet count—thrombocytopenia
- 20 minutes whole blood clotting time—may be prolonged
- Take 2 mL blood in glass tube and keep it undisturbed for 20 min—if not clotted, means coagulopathy
- Prothrombin time (PT)/activated partial thromboplastin time (APTT)—prolonged
- Fibrin degradation products (FDP)/D-dimer-increased in DIC
- Urine examination for proteinuria/RBC/hemoglobinuria/myoglobinuria
- Biochemistry for serum creatinine/urea/potassium—for renal failure
- Serum CK—for rhabdomyolysis
- Oxygen saturation/arterial blood gas (ABG)—type 2 respiratory failure

Management

Initial Management

- Removing the patient from the surroundings. Reassure the patient. 70% of snake bites are non-venomous,
- If possible, identify the snake but only if it does not delay patient transportation.
- Remove all tight fitting clothes, jewellery and footwear.
- Immobilizing the part by using a splint.
- Transport the person to the nearest medical facility
- Do not allow the patient to walk as this can cause increased blood pumped into the heart from the extremities which could contribute to spreading of the venom.

Things to avoid:

- Tourniquets should not be tied.
- In case a patient is received with a tourniquet, it should be removed slowly and not all at once.
- Avoid making incisions over the bite site.
- Avoid cleaning the bite site with chemicals.

Initial management in hospital:

Check vitals:

- Correct hypotension
- Intubate and ventilate for respiratory paralysis

Anti-snake venom administration: Specific treatment

India polyvalent ASV is effective against all the four common species

- Russell's viper, common cobra, common krait, saw-scaled viper.
- Response to ASV is present in all except hump-nosed viper bites.

Indications for ASV administration:

- Coagulopathy
- Neurotoxicity
- Severe local reaction involving more than half the affected limb or spreading rapidly.
- Severe abdomen pain and vomiting.
- Cardiovascular instability like arrhythmias, hypotension.

Administration of ASV

Start immediately for best effect. Can be started at any time after the bite. Even after one week if signs of envenomation are present.

Dose requirement:

- Purely localized swelling—no role of ASV
- If rapidly progressive swelling—start ASV
- Local reaction severe/hematological or neurological effects—8–16 vials, maximum dose—up to 50 vials

NEUROPARALYTIC BITE

- A usual initial dose of 10 vials is given in 500 mL 5% dextrose or saline over 30 min.
- If no improvement in 1 hour,10 more vials can be repeated again in the same way.

VASCULOTOXIC BITE

1. Low dose infusion method
   - 10 vials (Russel)/6 vials (saw scaled) over 30 min infusion
   - Followed by 2 vials 6th hourly over 30 min infusion
   - Endpoint—till clotting time is normal or 3 days (whichever is earlier)
2. High dose bolus method
   - 10 vials over 30 min
   - Followed by 6 vials bolus 6th hourly
   - Endpoint—till clotting time is normal or local swelling subsides (whichever is earlier)

There is *no requirement of a test dose.*

- Give 25 mg of pheniramine IV and 100 mg hydrocortisone IV prior to the ASV administration.
- Patients must be observed for hypotension, rashes, respiratory distress.
- No contraindication in pregnancy.
- Children require higher dose.

Monitoring and dose adjustment: According to toxicity—no fixed dose

- Hematotoxicity, repeat coagulation profile (PT/APTT) every 6 hours and ASV can be repeated if the profile is still deranged.
- For neurotoxicity, patients are observed for improvement of neurological symptoms.
- Up to 50 vials of ASV can be administered to the patient.

- In case of neurotoxicity.
  - Neostigmine can be given at 0.5–2 mg IV along with atropine 0.6 mg IV.
  - If neurological improvement occurs, it should be continued as follows:
    - Every 30 min for 5 doses
    - Then at 1 hr, 2 hr, 6 hr and 12 hr

Reaction to ASV: Treat as anaphylactic shock,

Additional Management

Local reaction:

- Inj TT 0.5 cc IM
- For cellulitis of affected limb, limb elevation along with glycerine magnesium sulphate dressing
- Appropriate IV antibiotics (amoxycillin and clavulanic acid/piperacillin tazobactum) for severe cellulitis after drawing blood cultures.
- Surgical consultation: Fasciotomy/debridement.

Pain

- Inj tramadol 50 mg IV 8th hourly
- Chymotrypsin + serratiopeptidase
- Avoid NSAIDS as they can cause bleeding and renal dysfunction

Supportive care

- For bleeding: FFP/packed cells
- Shock: IV fluids and inotropes
- Renal failure: Dialysis
- Respiratory paralysis: Intubate and ventilate

Prognosis

Early detection of envenomation and early ASV if indicated is essential in treatment of snake bite. Identification of the snake is also important in order to make a diagnosis of the type of bite.

Chapter 82

Scorpion Sting

- Mesobuthus tamulus—Indian red scorpion.

Clinical Features

- Clinical presentations may vary between scorpion species
  - *Centruroides* and *Parabuthus* species cause neuromuscular issues
  - *Buthus, Mesobuthus*, and *Androctonus* species cause life-threatening cardiovascular effects
- Onset of symptoms: In a few minutes
- Local features: Pain, erythema, necrotic ulceration
- Mixed autonomic dysfunction:
  - Parasympathetic: Bradycardia, hypotension, increased urination, hypersalivation, bronchoconstriction, vomiting, diarrhea and priapism
  - Sympathetic: Tachycardia, hypertension, profuse sweating and urinary retention.

Complications

- Cardiovascular complications: Pulmonary edema, ventricular arrhythmias and myocarditis.
- Respiratory failure
- Neurological manifestations: Paralysis, seizures and coma
- Acute kidney injury
- Rhabdomyolysis
- Acute pancreatitis
- Anaphylaxis to the venom

Investigations

- CBC and peripheral smear-leukocytosis and hemolysis, serum electrolytes-hyperkalemia, hyperglycemia, elevation of amylase, cardiac enzymes and liver transaminases, CK levels and urine analysis.

Treatment

- Supportive therapy
  - Pain management
- NSAIDs/paracetamol/opioids

- Cold compression
- Infiltration of sting site with local anesthetic/regional nerve block
  - Local wound care
  - Tetanus prophylaxis
  - Bronchospasm: Salbutamol
  - Anaphylaxis
    - Adrenaline
    - Hydrocortisone
  - Agitation
    - Benzodiazepines and haloperidol
  - Maintain normal fluid and electrolyte balance, but avoid fluid overload
- Anti-scorpion venom
  - Monovalent anti-scorpion venom serum F(ab)2 against mesobuthis tamulus
  - Single 30 mL dose is added to 100 mL normal saline and infused intravenously over 30 minutes, irrespective of the patients age
  - Risk of hypersensitivity present. Hence monitor the patient for at least 24 hours following anti-scorpion venom treatment.
- **Prazosin:**
  - Dose: 0.5 mg (30 microg/kg/dose) at 3 hourly intervals
  - Counteracts the sympathetic storm and prevents cardiotoxicity

Table 78.1: Bawaskar's Protocol for scorpion sting

Stage	Timing	Manifestations	Treatment
I	0–4 hours	Sweating, salivation, mydriasis, priapism, hypertension, cold extremities	Anti-scorpion venom + prazosin
II	4–6 hours	Hypertension, tachycardia, cold extremities	Anti-scorpion venom + Prazosin
III	6–10 hours	Cold extremities, tachycardia, hypotension, pulmonary edema	Anti-scorpion venom + prazosin + dobutamine + assisted ventilation
IV	0–6 hours	Massive pulmonary edema	Anti-scorpion venom + nitroglycerine + assisted ventilation
V	>12 hours	Warm shock: Tachycardia, hypotension, warm extremities, pulmonary edema	Dobutamine

Chapter

83

Animal Bite

- The main concern with animal bites is the possibility of rabies which has almost 100% fatality.
- All patients with animal bites should receive a rabies vaccine, irrespective of the animal showing symptoms of rabies. Asymptomatic animals can transmit rabies.
- History about the animal:
  - Whether it was domesticated or wild.
  - Wild animals including raccoons, bats, squirrels, monkeys, etc.
  - Domesticated animals including dogs (most common), cats and even cattle
  - Whether the bite was provoked or not.
  - The animal at time might be asymptomatic—so follow up history is important
- Using history and examination categorize the exposure to determine further management.

WHO CLASSIFICATION OF DOG BITE

Category of exposure	Description of the wound	Post exposure prophylaxis (PEP)
Category I	Touching or feeding animals, licks on intact skin, contact of intact skin with secretions or excretions of animal	No PEP required
Category II	Nibbling of uncovered skin, minor scratches or abrasions without bleeding	Vaccination
Category III	• Single or multiple transdermal bites with bleeding or scratches. • Licks on broken skin, exposure of mucosal surfaces to saliva. • All wounds over the face and head. • All wild animal bites are class III	Vaccination + immunoglobulin

Management

1. Wound Management

- Immediate washing and flushing wound for 15 minutes with soap and water, or water alone
- Then clean with povidone iodine solution

- In case of bleeding wounds, simple dressing can be applied over the wound
- Postpone suturing if possible; if suturing is necessary it should be done only after giving immunoglobulins locally

2. Rabies Vaccination

- For category I and II exposures
- The vaccination series may be discontinued if the biting dog is domesticated, and is alive after ten days of observation. ***This rule cannot be applied to other animal bites or street dogs.***
- In the process, if the patient has received at least three doses of rabies vaccine, and they can skip the day 14 dose, and take one dose on day 28.
- Also this is applicable only for the IM regimen, not the intradermal one.

Intramuscular route

i. The 5 dose intramuscular regime: (1-1-1-1-1)
   - One dose of the vaccine should be administered on days 0, 3, 7, 14 and 28
   - Given in the deltoid region for adults, or for young children, into the antero-lateral area of the thigh muscle.

ii. The 2-1-1 regimen: (2-0-1-0-1)
   - Two doses are given on day 0 in the deltoid muscle, right and left arm
   - An additional one dose is administered in the deltoid muscle on day 7 and day 21

Intramuscular route is cost effective as a smaller amount is required to be injected. It is provided free of cost in government institutes

i. The 2-site intradermal method: (2-2-2-0-2)
   - Dose: 0.1 mL
   - One dose is given intradermally at two different sites
   - Usually administered in the deltoid muscle on the left and right upper arm and suprascapular area
   - Given on days 0, 3, 7 and 28.

For individuals who have been previously vaccinated (if duration from completed course >3 months):

- 1-site ID on days 0 and 3; or
- 4-sites ID on day 0; over right and left deltoid, thigh or suprascapular areas), or
- 1-site IM on days 0 and 3

This is also only for category II and III exposures. If the patient has completed the course in the last three months, only wound management is sufficient.

Note

There are no contraindications to rabies vaccination like pregnancy, lactation, old age or infancy.

3. Rabies immunoglobulins (RIG) passive immunization

- Only for category III exposures
- Administered only once, as soon as possible after the initiation of PEP and not beyond day 7 after the first dose of vaccine. (need not be given in previously immunized individuals.)

- Two types of RIG are available—human RIG and equine RIG. Both are equally effective.
- RIG maximum doses—human RIG (hRIG) 20 IU/kg and equine RIG (eRIG) 40 IU/kg.
- eRIG being cheaper is more widely available. It comes as a 5 mL vial equivalent to 1500 IU in one vial. hRIG comes as a vial of 2.5 mL containing 100 IU per vial.
- Infiltrate as much as possible into the wound using an insulin syringe.
- The remaining dose of RIG need not be injected at a distance as recommended previously. It can be stored in the refrigerator and used for another patient.

4. Antibiotics

- Prophylactic antibiotics to be given only if there is clinical evidence of infected wound, deep wounds or immunocompromised individuals.
- Empirically amoxicillin clavulanate 1 g bd can be started
- In case of penicillin allergy, clindamycin 300 mg bd or doxycycline 100 mg bd can be started.

5. Tetanus Toxoid (TT) and tetanus human immunoglobulins (TIG)

- Dose of TIG: 250 units intramuscularly at a different site than tetanus toxoid
- Dose of TT: 0.5 mL given intramuscularly

Previous doses of tetanus toxoid	**Clean and minor wounds**		**All other wounds**	
<3 doses or unknown	TT to be given	No TIG required	TT to be given	TIG required
>3 doses	TT to be given only if last dose given ≥10 years ago	No TIG required	TT to be given only if last dose given ≥5 years ago	No TIG required

Section

10

Miscellaneous

Chapter

84

Tumor Lysis Syndrome

- Tumor lysis syndrome (TLS) is an oncological emergency.
- It is caused by destruction of a large number of rapidly proliferating neoplastic cells.
- Commonly in aggressive malignancies such as lymphomas), acute lymphoblastic leukemia and rarely in solid tumors.

It is characterized by **biochemical abnormalities:**

- Hyperuricemia
- Hyperkalemia
- Hyperphosphatemia
- Hypocalcemia
- Acute kidney injury (AKI) and acidosis.

Cairo-Bishop definition for diagnosis of TLS

Laboratory TLS is defined as two or more abnormal values, **within 3 days before or 7 days after initiation of chemotherapy,** in the setting of adequate hydration and use of hypouricemic agent.

Clinical TLS is defined as laboratory TLS plus one or more of the clinical signs.

Laboratory TLS	Clinical TLS
Uric acid > 8 mg/dL	AKI (defined as creatinine >1.5 × ULN)
Potassium >6 mEq/dL	Cardiac arrhythmias
Phosphorus >4.6 mg/dL	Seizure, tetany, or other symptomatic hypocalcemia
Calcium < 7 mg/dL	

Clinical Features

- Nausea, vomiting, diarrhea, lethargy
- Hematuria
- Muscle cramps, tetany
- Cardiac arrhythmia, seizures and sudden death

Other Investigations Needed

- LDH—to assess the tumor burden
- ECG to detect arrhythmias

Management

Prophylaxis and prevention of TLS includes hydration and addition of hypouricemic agents.

Risk Stratification

Low risk	Intermediate risk	High risk
Most solid tumors	Small cell lung cancer	Burkitt lymphoma
Multiple myeloma and CLL	CLL started on chemotherapy	AML with TLC >100,000
Hodgkin's lymphoma		DLBCL

Hydration

- IV hydration with NS or RL: 2 L/m^2. It is the cornerstone of prevention and management of TLS.
- Diuretics: Frusemide is the diuretic of choice.

Electrolyte Imbalance

- For **hyperuricemia:**
  1. Allopurinol (inhibitor of xanthine oxidase reducing production of uric acid)
     - dose—10 mg/kg/day in 3 divided doses (max dose of 800 mg per day)
     - In renal failure—50% reduction in dose
     - IV preparation available
  2. Febuxostat: Selective inhibitor of xanthine oxidase
     - Dose—started at 40 mg and increased to maximum of 120 mg/day
     - No dose adjustment in renal failure
  3. Rasburicase
     - Recombinant urate oxidase
     - Dose of 0.2 mg/kg once daily for 5–7 days IV
     - Safe in renal failure
     - Contraindicated in patients with G6PD deficiency
- **Hyperkalemia:** Treat with potassium lowering agents
- **Hypocalcemia:** Calcium gluconate can be given in case arrhythmias are present
- **Hyperphosphatemia:** Renal replacement therapy if calcium phosphorus product is >70.
- Indications for renal replacement
  - Severe oliguria or anuria
  - Symptomatic fluid overload state, example—pulmonary edema
  - Persistent hyperkalemia
  - Symptomatic hypocalcemia
  - Calcium phosphate product ≥70 mg^2/dL^2

Chapter

85

Drowning

Nonfatal drowning generally is defined as survival, at least temporarily, after suffocation by submersion in a liquid medium.

Risk factors for drowning

- Inability to swim/trauma
- Seizure disorder/alcohol intake/drug use
- Hypothermia/cardiac arrhythmia

Effects of drowning

Pulmonary

- Aspirated water washes out surfactant causing acute respiratory distress syndrome
- Decreased lung compliance
- Ventilation–perfusion mismatching
- Chest X-ray can be normal, localized, perihilar or diffuse pulmonary edema.

Neurological

- Hypoxic neuronal damage
- Cerebral edema/raised ICT

Cardiovascular

- Arrhythmias can be secondary to hypothermia or hypoxia.
- Most common include sinus tachycardia, sinus bradycardia, atrial fibrillation

Renal

- Hypoxic acute tubular necrosis can occur in near fatal drowning.

Management

Immediate prehospital management

- Immediate resuscitation by bystanders can improve outcome in drowning.
- Rescue breathing should start as soon as a stable surface is reached.
- Pulse should be assessed and CPR should be initiated.

Cervical collars are not mandatory unless there are signs of spine injury or mechanism of drowning is suggestive of the same (diving accident)

In hospital emergency management

- Trauma assessment to look for other injuries (including cervical spine injuries)
- Wet clothes should be removed and warming blankets should be applied.

Inpatient management

1. **Neurological injuries**—goal is to prevent secondary neurological injuries due to ischemia, cerebral edema, hypotension, electrolyte imbalance.
    - Elevation of head end at 30 degrees.
    - Diuretics to decrease cerebral edema, titrated so as to not cause hypotension.
    - Prevent seizures by using non-sedative antiepileptics like phenytoin.
    - Avoid neuromuscular blockers.
    - Prevent hypo- and hyperglycemia. Maintain a sugar level of 180–200 mg/dL
    - Hyperventilation can be tried in patients with imminent threat of herniation. Prolonged hyperventilation should be avoided as it causes vasoconstriction and decreased cerebral blood flow.
2. Respiratory
    - Bronchospasm is common and should be treated with nebulization.
    - Antibiotics are indicated in case chest X-ray shows features of consolidation. Pseudomonas should be covered in this case.
    - Mechanical ventilation if indicated:
        - If SPO_2 is <90 or pO_2 is <60 on high flow oxygen
        - Drowsy patient
        - In patients on non-invasive ventilation, saturation is to be maintained above 94%
    - ECMO has been tried in a few case series but there is not too much evidence supporting its use.
    - Use of exogenous surfactant: Has been tried.
3. Cardiac arrhythmias: Treat as per standard guidelines.

The following are associated with poor prognosis in drowning

- Duration of submersion >5 minutes (most critical factor)
- Time to effective basic life support >10 minutes
- Resuscitation duration >25 minutes
- Age >14 years
- Glasgow Coma Scale <5 (i.e. comatose)
- Persistent apnea and requirement of cardiopulmonary resuscitation in the emergency department
- Arterial blood pH <7.1 upon presentation

Chapter

86

Near Hanging

- Refers to survivors of an attempted hanging
- Note:
  - Partial hanging: Some part of the body touches the floor
  - Complete hanging: Full suspension of the body above the ground
- May be suicidal/homicidal/accidental

Clinical features and complications

- Laryngeal injury
- Injury to vascular structures:
  - Jugular vein (most common) > carotid artery > vertebral artery (rare)
  - Arterial and venous obstruction > stagnant cerebral hypoxia
  - Tardieu's spots (facial petechiae) and subconjunctival hemorrhages: Due to venous hypertension
  - Compression of the carotid bodies > reflex bradycardia
- CNS complications:
    - Status epilepticus
    - Cerebral edema
    - Subarachnoid hemorrhage
    - Upper cervical cord injury
    - Hypoxic-ischemic brain injury
- Pulmonary complications:
  - Aspiration pneumonia/ARDS
  - Pulmonary edema
    - Neurogenic—due to centrally mediated, massive sympathetic discharge
    - Postobstructive—generation of large, negative intrathoracic pressures, due to attempted inspiration in the presence of upper airway obstruction;
    - Cardiogenic—as a result of hanging-associated takotsubo cardiomyopathy

Investigations

- Routine lab investigations including ABG
- X-ray—cervical spine lateral view/CT neck
- CT brain: Detection of subarachnoid hemorrhage/cerebral edema/cerebral infarction
- CT/MRI scanning of the cervical cord: In patients with features of upper cord injury

Management

- Immediate relief of suspension and removal of the ligature
- Cervical spine (C-spine) immobilization
- Airway and breathing—
  - If the patient is spontaneously breathing, administer high-flow oxygen
  - If inadequate:
    - Bag and mask ventilation
    - Rapid-sequence endotracheal intubation: If the bag and mask ventilation is inadequate for ventilating the patient
    - In-line immobilization of the cervical spine should be performed during intubation and excessive motion of head and neck avoided
  - Mechanical ventilation
    - Positive pressure ventilation for pulmonary edema and ARDS
- Management of cerebral edema
  - 30 degree head up position
  - Hyperventilation (target $PaCO_2$: 30–35 mmHg)
  - Role of mannitol, diuretics, anticonvulsants and corticosteroids—controversial
- Resuscitation as per BLS/ACLS protocol if the patient is unresponsive

Chapter

87 HIV and Hepatitis B—Postexposure Prophylaxis for Healthcare Workers

Risk of infection

The risk of transmission following

- Percutaneous exposure—0.23%
- Mucous membrane exposure—0.09%
- Perinatal—15–30%
- Sexual contact—0.1 to 1%

Investigations for HIV antibody after exposure

- 1st sample: Immediately after exposure,
- 2nd: 6 weeks later
- 3rd: 12 weeks later
- Final test: 6 months after exposure
- HIV 1&2 RNA copies by PCR of the patient, if possible, to know the viral load.

Management

Local measures

- Thorough cleaning with soap for skin exposures, alcohol-based solution for small wounds and punctures.
- In case of mucosal surface exposure, flush the area with copious amount of water
- Do not place the pricked finger into the mouth reflexively
- Do not squeeze blood from wound
- Counselling—prior to testing
- Advice on protected sex for next 6 months, till HIV negative status is confirmed.

To start antiretroviral drug combination as early as possible

- Preferably within 2 hours of exposure (within 72 hours at most)
- Regimens: First dose—stat
  - Tenofovir 300 mg (TDF) + lamivudine 300 mg + efavirenz 600 mg, or
  - Tenofovir 300 mg (TDF) + emtricitabine 200 mg + dolutegravir 50 mg
- Subsequent doses should be taken at night, 2–3 hours after food. Avoid fatty food at dinner
- If efavirenz is not tolerated, then combination of tenofovir + lamivudine + protease inhibitor (atazanavir or lopinavir) can be used after expert consult.

Follow up:
- To monitor CBP while on above drugs
- Duration of treatment is 4 weeks

Annexure 1: HIV Exposure Code

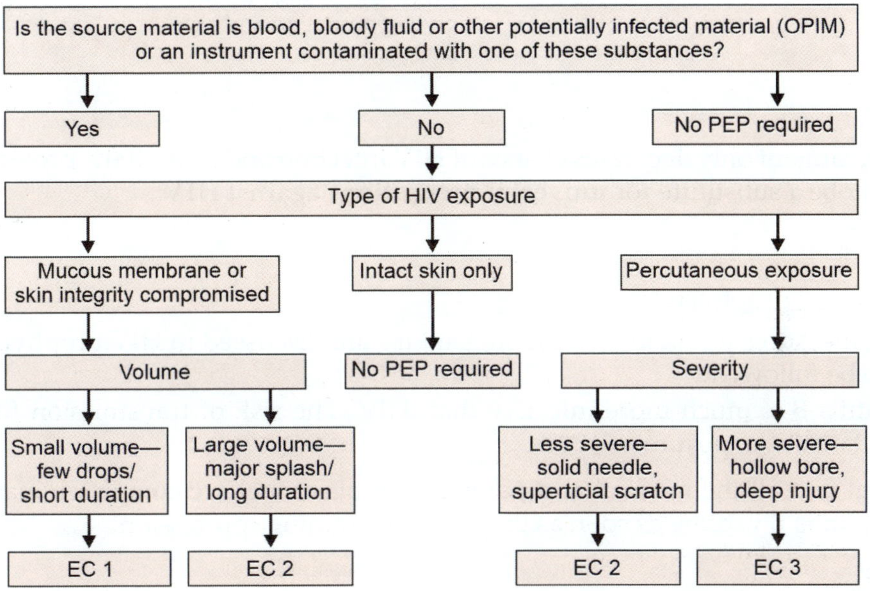

Annexure 2: HIV Source Code

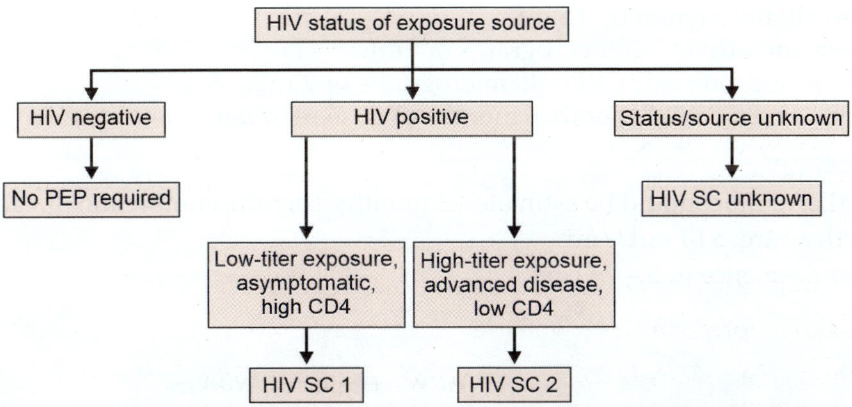

Exposure codes	HIV source code	PEP recommendations	Duration
1	1	Not warranted	28 days
1	2	Recommended	
2	1		
2	2		

Contd.

Contd.

Exposure codes	HIV source code	PEP recommendations	Duration
3	1 or 2		
2/3	Unknown	Consider PEP, if HIV prevalence is high in the given population and risk categorisation	

Note

Above treatment only decreases chance of HIV infection and is not 100% protective and can never be a substitute for **universal precautions against HIV**.

HEPATITIS B PROPHYLAXIS

Postexposure prophylaxis:

- Local measures following needle stick injury are discussed in HIV prophylaxis and are to be followed.
- Hepatitis B is much more infective than HIV. The risk of transmission following percutaneous exposure—6–30%

It is ideal that all the medical and paramedical personnel are completely vaccinated with hepatitis B vaccine as soon as they join the training/profession.

Note

Pregnancy is not a contraindication to vaccination.

Hepatitis B vaccine (DNA recombinant) IM in deltoid region

a. Infants—10 microgram or 0.5 mL
b. Children and adults—20 micrograms or 1mL.
c. Immunocompromised/CRF—40 micrograms or 2 mL.
Vaccination given on 0, 1 month, 6 months (3 dose regimen)

High risk persons

- Anti HBsAg titer should be estimated 3 months after the completion of vaccination.
- Protective titre: >10 mIU/mL.
- Booster dose once in 5 – 7 years.

Postexposure Prophylaxis

	HCW—Healthcare Workers		
Source	Unvaccinated or incomplete vaccination	Vaccinated	
		Anti-HBs > 10	Anti HBs < 10
HbsAg positive or unknown status	1 dose of HBIG + 1 dose of Hep B vaccine + complete the full course	PEP not necessary	1 dose of HBIG + 1 dose of Hep B vaccine + complete the full course
HbsAg negative	1 dose of Hep B vaccine + complete the full course	PEP Not Necessary	Single Hep B vaccine dose, repeat anti-HBs testing 1–2 months later. If <10—complete the full course

Index